MINDFULNES

PENDU~~~

The ultimate antidote to overthinking

Table of Contents

Anthony Talmage

Dowse [1] |douz| - To search for or discover something by intuition or sixth sense: *water is easy to dowse for; he dowsed a spiral of energy on the stone.* To search for underground water, minerals, etc., using a divining rod; to divine.

Mindfulness - A mental state achieved by focusing one's awareness on the present moment, while calmly acknowledging and accepting one's feelings, thoughts, and bodily sensations. Used as a therapeutic technique.

FOREWORD

Mindfulness And The Pendulum is not just a guide to Dowsing or Mindfulness; it's an invitation to embark on a journey of self-discovery, fueled by your unique intuition. By embracing the power of Dowsing practice, which you're going to learn all about, you can cultivate a deeper connection to yourself, the world around you, and the wisdom that lies within. This, in turn, will unlock a portal to a unique immersive Mindfulness.

And remember, Dowsing is a journey, not a destination. Embrace the practice, trust your intuition, and allow yourself to be guided on a path to greater Mindfulness and a life lived to the full.

CONTENTS

PREFACE

The twin topics of Dowsing and Mindfulness can be complex and certainly deserve a detailed examination. However, the basics are an important starting point and, hopefully, knowing them should lead naturally to a desire for the more challenging exposition which we'll move onto together. To offer the best of both worlds, I have divided this book into four distinct sections.

Part 1 is an overview of Dowsing and Mindfulness so we can see the context of our mission, Part 2 takes us on a deeper dive into the fascinating art of Dowsing. In Part 3 we look at Mindfulness and its techniques and Part 4, the anchor of this book, is how Dowsing and Mindfulness can work together to provide a unique kind of meditation to help protect us from a world that sometimes appears to be slipping into a collective insanity.

PART 1
Chapter 1

WELCOME TO YOUR INNER COMPASS

In this section, we dive into the mysterious and fascinating world of Dowsing, exploring common myths and discovering how this ancient skill has practical applications in today's world. Through gripping real-life stories—like the tale of George Applegate finding water in the drought-ridden Australian outback, and the experiences of everyday people like Walter Sehnert, who used Dowsing to find water, oil, and lost objects—you'll see that Dowsing is far more than just a superstition. It's a skill and a skill anyone can develop.

But this part isn't just about Dowsing. After exploring its incredible potential, we introduce Mindfulness and begin to lay the foundations for how these two powerful practices can work together. We learn the basics of Mindfulness, a modern approach to calming the mind and staying present, helping us manage stress and focus on the moment at hand. Together, Dowsing and Mindfulness can enhance our intuitive abilities and sharpen our awareness, opening doors to self-discovery and practical insight.

By the end of Part 1, we'll be ready to explore how these two seemingly unrelated practices—one ancient and the other modern—are perfect companions, and how integrating them can lead to greater self-awareness, clarity, and balance in our daily lives.

Chapter 2

DOWSING DOESN'T WORK - IT'S ALL JUST WISHFUL THINKING

(Oh No it isn't!)

The Australian outback shimmered under a relentless sun. The land, once a tapestry of vibrant greens and golds, had surrendered to a five-year drought. Waterholes were now dusty craters, and the lifeblood of the outback—cattle and sheep stations—teetered on the brink of extinction. Hope had become a scarce commodity, as precious as the elusive rain.

That's when a glimmer of hope arrived in the form of George Applegate, a wiry Englishman with a reputation as a miracle worker. Scoffed at by some as a "water witch," Applegate was a dowser, a man who claimed to locate hidden water with the help of a simple forked stick cut from a hazel tree. Despite their skepticism, the farmers' desperation had trumped their customary practicality, and they had pooled their resources to bring Applegate nearly 10,000 miles to work his magic.

Applegate, more comfortable in wellingtons than holding a briefcase, surveyed the parched landscape with a practiced eye. Ignoring the whispers of doubt that followed him, he began his work. Days blurred one into another as he traversed the cracked earth, the hazel twig clutched tightly in his hands, hovering like a bird of prey seeking its victim. The farmers watched, a mixture of hope and resignation etched on their faces.

Then, on a day so hot the air shimmered like a mirage, Applegate stopped dead in his tracks. The hazel twig, usually inert, twitched violently in his grasp. His audience gasped. Applegate's weathered face broke into a wide grin.

"Water," he declared, his voice hoarse with excitement. Using the end of his Dowsing instrument as a pointer, he added, "There's a sizeable body of water right here. The bad news is, it's over a quarter of a mile down."

Disbelief alternated with hope in the farmers' eyes. They had drilled in this area before, with no success. But maybe they just hadn't gone deep enough. It was going to be a big risk, but there was something about Applegate's conviction and the way the twig danced in his hand that rekindled a spark of belief.

With renewed purpose, they hired drilling equipment, costing thousands of dollars a day. Was this going to be the last desperate act that would lead to bankruptcy, or would their final throw of the dice pay off? For days, the drill bit burrowed deeper into the earth. Finally, a cheer erupted—water! Could it be? Or was this another mirage? After a few spluttering squirts, a crystal-clear spout surged from the hole. George had achieved the seemingly miraculous.

Later tests revealed that Applegate had tapped into a 10,000-year-old aquifer, a hidden oasis that had remained undiscovered for millennia. The drought had finally been vanquished, the land drank deeply, and the once-parched outback bloomed again.

George Applegate, the dowser who defied skepticism with a hazel twig, became a legend whispered across the vast expanse of Australia—a symbol of hope rekindled in the face of despair.

Quite a yarn, eh? And it's all true. George was the first to insist that he was nothing special. He wasn't gifted. Anyone can do what he did if they apply themselves to learning the skills. And this includes you, reading this now. Dowsing is a special way of tapping into our sixth sense, and that's what you and I will be learning as we embark on this journey of discovery together.

Chapter 3

Not quite convinced? Here's a story printed in the McCook Gazette, Nebraska: WALTER'S WONDERFUL WITCHING WAND

My dad, Walter Sehnert, was a dowser—a diviner—a witcher of water. I think he had always had an interest in locating water using a forked stick, but it was only after he retired from the bakery that he pursued the ancient art of Dowsing with real passion. In his later years, he and Ella, my stepmother, attended the International Dowsers Convention at Danville, Vermont, at least twice, and an International Convention in California, in addition to numerous regional meetings throughout the Midwest, which were devoted to the various ways one could use divining rods.

Dowsing for objects—most commonly water—has been around since ancient times and has always been greeted with skepticism. There seem to be two points of view when it comes to Dowsing:

1. Those who believe in it feel that, using one of several types of divining devices, they can detect emanations of energy, radiations, or vibrations caused by the thing they are Dowsing for.

2. Many people, however, believe the dowser is under the influence of suggestion or expectation, which affects involuntary and unconscious motor behavior, causing the divining device to move.

Whether you swear by Dowsing or swear at it, the fact is that dowsers all over the world regularly use divining instruments to find water and pinpoint the best location for a new well. Some oil exploration teams, even with the sophisticated scientific methods now available, still use the services of a dowser to choose the exact spot to drill on an oil lease property. In Germany, builders are required to have a dowser inspect a building site for noxious rays (which might contaminate the site) before they are issued a building permit.

My dad was most comfortable Dowsing for water, which he did often on his own farm. He also helped farmers in northeast Nebraska find the best location for a new well. He never charged for his service. He was realistic enough to know that he would not always be successful and didn't want to take responsibility in case of failure.

The ability to dowse seems to be a gift (or perhaps a skill?) that a person either has or hasn't. One can learn various techniques, but to be successful, one really needs to believe in the process. Dad tried to help me dowse on a number of occasions. I was a hopeless case. So was Ella, my stepmother. When they attended the big Dowsers' Convention in Danville, Dad and Ella always attended the Dowsers' School to learn new techniques and practice in a field that had been "salted" with various artifacts. After attending the school for a second year, the instructor took Ella aside and gently suggested she take up another hobby.

"Some folks just don't have the gift," he told her as kindly as he could. I understood just how she felt. Dowsing did not come easily for me either.

Dad and Ella enjoyed the conventions in Danville, where they formed friendships with like-minded people from every state and even foreign countries. They assumed they would find a similar atmosphere at the Dowsers' Convention in Los Angeles. They were wrong. When they returned from that trip, they were quite shaken. While the Danville dowsers had concentrated on finding water, oil, and hidden objects, with a bit of map Dowsing, the Los Angeles dowsers leaned toward the occult and contacting spirits and "spooky stuff." They never returned to California for another dowsers meeting.

At the RV park in Texas, where they wintered for many years, Dad became something of a celebrity when he successfully advised the park maintenance crew on locating a buried water pipe. They knew it was leaking, but they had no idea where to dig. His instructions were exact and saved the park considerable expense.

It was at this park that I witnessed a demonstration that convinced me there must be something to this business of Dowsing. One day, the fellow who delivered propane to the park patrons stopped to fill Dad's tanks. Dad had two tanks and instructed the fellow to fill one of them. When asked about the second, Dad told him that it was nearly full.

"How do you know it's full? The gauge is broken," the fellow said.

"I know because I dowsed it with my divining rod," Dad replied.

The fellow laughed, clearly an unbeliever. He covered the dial on his propane truck with his hand.

"OK, if that stick of yours is so smart, tell me how much propane I've got in my big tank."

Dad waved his wand up and down over the tank and pointed to a spot about a third of the way up the tank.

"Well, I'll be d——d, if that doesn't beat all!" the fellow muttered as he drove away. The dial on the truck's tank indicated exactly one-third full.

Dowsing for More Than Water

People were always trying to get Dad to dowse for things besides water, which he was often reluctant to do. However, he often went along with his friends' requests. One fellow was sure there was gold on his land, at a place where water bubbled to the surface, creating two streams, one flowing north to the Niobrara River, the other flowing south to the Elkhorn. Dad dowsed the site, and the results were negative—no gold. The gold-colored film on the water turned out to be iron oxide.

Another lady was convinced there was oil on her land. Dad agreed that it appeared to be so, though he could only get a general reading of oil over her entire farm. Subsequent drilling by oil companies found significant amounts of oil, and eventually, producing wells were established on each quarter of her land.

On one occasion, the Norfolk, Nebraska, police contacted Dad for help in finding a teenage girl who had been missing for several weeks. Dad attached her picture to his wand and swung a pendulum over a map of Nebraska. He was unable to pinpoint a location, but when asked specific questions, the pendulum indicated that the girl was dead. Later, the girl's body was found buried in a shallow grave. That experience unnerved Dad, and he vowed never to get involved in searching for missing persons again. He kept that promise.

Each year, when Dad and Ella returned from the South, he had some sort of new tool for divining. One year, this tool was a wand with a spring attached to a pendulum. After supper one evening, he demonstrated his new gadget to the family, using it to locate coins hidden in the room. While he was engaged in this activity, my son Matt's friends stopped by to pick him up on their way to the movies.

Like all young fellows, they were intrigued by the performance, and each took a turn at "Dowsing." After a time, Dad mentioned that he could also measure a person's aura—a halo that surrounds one's body. By measuring the aura, one could detect weaknesses in a person's health.

"OK, Poppa," Matt said. "Measure Kent's aura. See what you can find."

Kent, a fine athlete and the quarterback on the football team, was in great physical shape. Dad had never met Kent before. Dad began his measurement of Kent's aura, starting at his side, below the waist, and moving up over his head and down the other side. The pendulum stayed about six inches away from his body.

"Wow, Kent," Dad said. "You've got a really strong aura. You must be in great shape." Just then, the pendulum swung abruptly in, striking Kent's body at his knee.

"Do you have knee problems, Kent?" Dad asked.

"Yeah," Kent replied. "I go in Monday for arthroscopic surgery."

There was a stunned silence for a long moment—and a new batch of believers in Walter's Wonderful Witching Wand.

Chapter 4

YES, BUT...

What is Dowsing?

Dowsing is an ancient practice used to locate underground water, minerals, lost objects, and even gain insights into personal questions by interpreting the movements of a Dowsing tool, such as a pendulum, L-rods, or a Y-rod. Dowsing works by connecting the dowser to subtle energies or information fields that are not typically accessible through the five senses.

How does Dowsing work?

The exact mechanism of Dowsing is not fully understood, but many believe that it taps into the dowser's subconscious mind or an energy field, sometimes referred to as the "universal mind" or "field of consciousness." When you ask a question while holding a Dowsing tool, your subconscious may guide the subtle movements of the tool to provide answers. Some theories suggest that Dowsing works by accessing the body's natural ability to perceive changes in energy fields.

What tools do dowsers use?

The most common Dowsing tools are:

• **Pendulums**: A weighted object, such as a crystal or metal, suspended on a chain or string.

• **L-Rods**: Two L-shaped rods, usually made of metal, held loosely in each hand.

• **Y-Rods (or forked sticks)**: A Y-shaped branch or metal rod, traditionally used for finding water.

• **Bobbers**: A flexible rod with a weight at the end, which bounces or "bobs" in response to questions.

Can anyone learn to dowse?

Yes, Dowsing is a skill that almost anyone can learn with practice. While some people may have a natural affinity for it, others can develop their Dowsing abilities over time. The key is to remain open-minded, practice regularly, and be patient as you learn to interpret the responses from your Dowsing tool.

How do I start Dowsing?

To start Dowsing, follow these basic steps:

1. **Choose a Dowsing tool**: Start with a pendulum, as it is easy for beginners to use.

2. **Relax and focus**: Find a quiet space where you won't be disturbed. Take a few deep breaths to center yourself.

3. **Ask clear questions**: Hold your pendulum and ask simple yes/no questions. Make sure your questions are specific and clear.

4. **Observe the movements**: Notice how the pendulum moves. For example, it might swing back and forth for "yes" and side to side for "no."

5. **Interpret the answers**: Over time, you'll learn to interpret the movements of your pendulum more accurately.

What kind of questions can I ask when Dowsing?

You can ask almost any type of question that can be answered with a "yes," "no," or sometimes "maybe." Examples include: "Is this the right decision for me?" "Should I meditate now?" "Is this the best place to plant this tree?" "Is this food beneficial for my health?"

How do I know if my Dowsing results are accurate?

Accuracy in Dowsing improves with practice. It's essential to be in a calm and neutral state of mind when Dowsing, as strong emotions or preconceived notions can influence the results. It's also helpful to validate your findings with real-world results when possible, such as checking if the water you dowsed for is actually present when digging.

Can Dowsing be used for more than just finding water?

Absolutely! While Dowsing is traditionally known for finding water, it can be used in various other ways, including:

Finding lost objects: Locating items such as keys, jewelry, or even pets
.

Health inquiries: Assessing the body's energy levels, identifying food sensitivities, or determining the best time to rest.

Spiritual guidance: Gaining insights into personal or spiritual questions, such as life direction or emotional well-being.

Space clearing: Identifying and clearing negative energies in your living space.

Is there any scientific evidence supporting Dowsing?

Dowsing remains controversial in the scientific community, and there is no widely accepted scientific explanation for how it works. Some studies have shown success in controlled Dowsing experiments, while others have not. However, many dowsers and practitioners report consistent and useful results, and Dowsing has been used successfully in various practical applications for centuries.

How can I improve my Dowsing skills?

Here are some tips for improving your Dowsing abilities:

• **Practice regularly**: Like any skill, Dowsing improves with regular practice.

• **Stay neutral**: Approach Dowsing without expectations or emotional attachments to the outcome.

• **Keep a journal**: Record your Dowsing questions, responses, and outcomes to track your progress and improve your accuracy.

- **Experiment**: Try Dowsing in different environments and with different questions to expand your experience.
- **Trust the process**: Trust that with time and practice, you will develop a stronger connection to your Dowsing tool and the information it provides.

What are some common mistakes to avoid when Dowsing?

- **Leading questions**: Avoid asking questions that suggest a particular answer, as this can influence the result.
- **Over-Dowsing**: Dowsing too frequently on the same issue can lead to confusion and inaccurate answers.
- **Ignoring your intuition**: While Dowsing tools are helpful, your intuition plays a crucial role in interpreting the results.
- **Being impatient**: Dowsing requires patience and practice; rushing the process can lead to frustration and inaccurate answers.

Can Dowsing be used to help others?

Yes, many dowsers use their skills to help others by finding lost objects, locating water, assessing health concerns, or providing spiritual guidance. However, it's important to approach Dowsing for others with care, ensuring that you have their permission and that you're in a neutral state of mind when doing so.

Is Dowsing related to psychic abilities?

Dowsing is often associated with psychic abilities because it involves accessing information beyond the five senses. Some believe that Dowsing taps into a form of intuition or extrasensory perception (ESP). Whether or not you consider it a psychic ability, Dowsing can enhance your connection to your inner guidance and intuition.

What should I do if I'm not getting any clear responses?

If your Dowsing tool isn't responding clearly, try the following:

- **Relax**: Take a few deep breaths and release any tension or expectations.
- **Rephrase the question**: Ensure your question is clear and straightforward.
- **Check your energy levels**: If you're tired or emotionally drained, take a break and return to Dowsing later.
- **Ground yourself**: Sometimes, grounding techniques like standing barefoot on the earth can help clear your energy and improve your connection with the Dowsing tool.

Can Dowsing be harmful or used for negative purposes?

Dowsing, like any tool, should be used with positive intentions and ethical considerations. It's important to use Dowsing to help and guide rather than to manipulate or harm others. Always approach Dowsing with respect, and be mindful of the potential impact of the information you receive.

Chapter 5

MINDFULNESS DOESN'T WORK –
IT'S JUST A NEW-AGE FAD
(Oh Yes it does, and Oh No it isn't)

A Journey from Anxiety to Peace - A personal story from Karen:

From as early as I can remember, anxiety was a constant companion in my life. Even as a young child, I was plagued by fears that seemed to overshadow every aspect of my existence. Going to sleep was the worst part of my day, filled with dread and an overwhelming sense of unease. My greatest wish was to stay by my mother's side, day and night, for that was the only place I felt somewhat safe.

School terrified me. The idea of being surrounded by a large group of children I didn't know was paralyzing. I was scared to be in a car with more than three people, consumed by the fear that the car might break down. Boats were out of the question; I was convinced they would sink. I couldn't bear to be left at home with a childminder, gripped by the fear that my mother might never come back.

These fears dominated my childhood. I constantly believed something terrible was going to happen—that I would get lost, have to go to the hospital, be separated from my mother and sister, endure immense pain, or even die. These catastrophic thoughts kept me in a state of high alert, where life itself felt overwhelmingly scary.

For nearly four decades, anxiety was an unpleasant and relentless companion. Although therapy during my childhood and later years helped reduce the severity of my anxiety, it never fully left me. Then, in 2008, at the age of 40, I was introduced to Mindfulness—a practice that would ultimately change my life.

Mindfulness didn't provide an instant cure, but it gave me something far more valuable: understanding. Through Mindfulness practice, I began to understand the roots of my anxiety and, more importantly, how to respond to it with compassion rather than fear.

My parents divorced when I was just two years old, and my mother raised my sister and me as a single mom, working full-time to provide for us. This meant we had to grow up quickly, learning to navigate life without the constant reassurance that everything was okay. While my mother did her best, her absence often left me feeling scared and unsafe. Mindfulness helped me see that my anxiety was a response to these early experiences, not a flaw in my character.

Transforming My Relationship with Stress

Mindfulness has made me more aware of my stress patterns. When anxiety sets in, a familiar narrative plays in my head: *"It's too much, I have too much work to do, I can't cope, I won't be able to do it."* These thoughts trigger my mind's alarm system, leading to physical tension, shallow breathing, and a cascade of stress reactions that affect my interactions with others.

In the past, this cycle of anxiety would spiral out of control, fueled by harsh self-criticism. I would beat myself up for being stressed, grumpy, or inefficient, which only added another layer of anxiety and stress. But Mindfulness opened my eyes to a crucial truth: harsh self-criticism is one of the most significant sources of stress and anxiety, and it can even lead to depression.

Seeing Things as They Are

Mindfulness has taught me to see things more clearly, without the distortions of anxiety and stress. Yes, I have work to do and deadlines to meet, but they are just that—work and deadlines. They don't define me, and they don't have to dictate my emotional state. This understanding, called primary experience, allows me to separate what is actually happening from the stories my mind creates about it—stories that often cause unnecessary pain.

Mindfulness is not just an idea; it's a practice. It requires daily commitment, faith, and perseverance. But the rewards are immense.

Practical Tools for Peace

When I feel stress or anxiety rising, I now have tools to bring myself back to the present moment. I notice my breath becoming shallow, my thoughts racing, and the tension building in my body. I take deeper breaths, allowing my breath to find its natural rhythm again, which helps my mind and body relax.

Mindfulness has transformed how I experience myself. It has helped me recognize my habitual ways of thinking and behaving—both helpful and unhelpful—and has enabled me to respond differently, with more kindness and compassion toward myself and others.

Living with Mindfulness

Today, anxiety still visits me, particularly in the early hours of the morning. I wake up with my heart racing and my mind filled with catastrophic thoughts. But now, I know what to do. I expand my in-breath and slow down my out-breath. I feel my body grounded on the mattress, noticing the sensations in my feet, legs, back, and head. I acknowledge the catastrophic thoughts and gently ask myself, "Is this true?" Ninety-nine percent of the time, the answer is no. I'm back in the present moment, able to calm down and return to sleep.

Mindfulness has given me back my life. It's not just an idea or a fleeting trend—it's a practice that requires dedication and patience. But the payoff is profound. It has transformed my relationship with anxiety and stress, and it has allowed me to live more fully, with greater peace and clarity.

If you're feeling doubtful about the benefits of Mindfulness, I encourage you to give it a try. It may not be an instant fix, but with time and practice, it can lead to deep and lasting change. Mindfulness has given me a new lease on life, and it can do the same for you.

Chapter 6

A CRAZY YEAR, THEN MINDFULNESS FOUND ME

Rebecca in the UK tells her Mindfulness Story:

It's true to say that I never went looking for Mindfulness, as such. It found me. It was back in 2019. I had settled back home in the Midlands after a crazy year of traveling as a freelance performing artist, and I was applying for a new job.

The position I was applying for was 'Healthy Living Officer' for deaf people. A doddle, I thought, given my knowledge and keen interest in nutrition and fitness. During the interview, my employer explained that a compulsory element of the position was that I must be willing to be trained as a Mindfulness practitioner.

I was asked if I knew anything about it. Mindfulness... hmm. Scrambling through my photographic memory, I recalled pages from a yoga book and began to waffle on about 'living in the moment,' and breathing techniques. In truth, I had no idea what I was talking about, but as my employer smiled back, I felt quietly confident that I'd got away with it.

I was offered the position in May and began my intensive training as a Mindfulness Practitioner just three months later. A tutor from Mindfulness Scotland flew down each week to deliver the sessions, and as I opened myself up to the course and practiced what I was learning, I found myself feeling extremely grateful for the opportunity to be immersed in Mindfulness.

Because in all honesty, I needed it.

One of the main reasons I settled back home and reduced all of my performing arts jobs was that at the young age of 22, I suffered a period of what I would call 'burnout.'

I had been pouring myself into four different jobs across the country, often traveling 300 miles a day, three days a week, and I was exhausted in every sense. I couldn't see it at the time, but I had been ignoring every possible sign my body had been giving me to slow down.

By being introduced to Mindfulness, I was able to see how I'd lived most of my life feeling constantly driven. Pushed on to achieve with 'no rest for the wicked,' I'd forgotten how to be gentle with myself. The concepts of compassion and self-acceptance were alien to me back then.

Similarly, I always felt unable to 'switch off.' When I wasn't working, I was lost in my head, planning, reflecting, or anticipating events yet to come. I never felt as though what I had or what I was doing was 'enough,' hence the overly ambitious and hardworking nature.

But what Mindfulness offered me was the ability to see clearly, for the first time, how I was really living my life. And in order to accept this and cultivate positive change, I learned how to go easy on myself and how to be my own best friend—something that I'd never considered before.

Back then, I thought life was supposed to be hard and tiring. I believed you only deserved good when you had achieved something remarkable or worked yourself to the ground. But Mindfulness showed me that thoughts are just thoughts. I no longer had to believe the flawed thoughts I had, or better still—be controlled by them. I could let them go and choose a different way.

Mindfulness also reminded me of the simple pleasures in life. I was introduced to the concept of a beginner's mind, a way of living that children naturally inhabit—so alert, curious, and engaged in the world around them. I felt as if I was seeing the world around me for the first time in a long time!

Nowadays, practicing Mindfulness can be as straightforward as allowing myself to quietly enjoy a cup of tea while abandoning all thoughts of work. I can draw myself out of my head and back into my body at any time, welcoming the peace and quiet that can always be found in the present moment.

I'm also much better now at diverting my attention away from frightening thoughts. I'm much more aware of when I'm wandering down 'what if' lane or indulging in negative reflections. And it's this awareness that gives me the option of choosing differently.

While it's true that Mindfulness is simple, it isn't always easy. Even now—after I've taught and spoken about Mindfulness for five years—there are still times where I 'forget.' But I am much better at remembering, and I'm much easier on myself. I'm only human, after all.

I would say the greatest gift Mindfulness has given me is self-compassion. By 'meeting myself at my own front door' and becoming my greatest friend, I've found that life feels a lot easier than it used to. I'm a lot kinder to myself, choosing kinder thoughts and behaving in a way that makes me feel good. I don't have to battle with my over-active mind or ambitions anymore. I can accept myself as I am, exactly as I am—in this moment.

I love sharing these mindful revelations with others, and I feel very blessed to work in an area that I believe in and have benefited from personally. Being fluent in sign language means I am also able to share these methods with Deaf and hard of hearing people and begin to make Mindfulness much more accessible.

Wishing all of you readers much love and self-compassion as you continue your own Mindfulness journey. Go easy on yourself.

A Personal Testimony from Charles:

At the age of forty, I was introduced to Mindfulness, and it transformed my life. For nearly four decades, anxiety had been my unwelcome companion, casting shadows over my days and nights. But through Mindfulness, I discovered a path to understanding and healing.

Mindfulness revealed to me the roots of my anxiety, stemming from a childhood marked by the absence of a stable parental presence. Raised by a single mother who juggled full-time work, my sister and I learned early to navigate life's challenges independently. Yet, beneath our façade of resilience lay deep-seated fears of inadequacy and insecurity.

The practice of Mindfulness became my refuge, guiding me to a place of self-awareness and compassion. It taught me to observe the patterns of stress and anxiety woven into the fabric of my existence. No longer did I succumb blindly to the torrent of worrisome thoughts or the physical manifestations of tension. Instead, I learned to recognize the triggers and respond with non-judgmental understanding.

Mindfulness illuminated the fallacy of self-criticism, revealing it as a source of unnecessary pressure and suffering. Through its lens, I saw the events of my life with clarity, distinguishing between primary experiences and the secondary narratives we weave around them. This newfound perspective liberated me from the grip of anxiety, allowing me to embrace each moment with equanimity.

While occasional bouts of anxiety still visit me, especially in the quiet hours of the morning, Mindfulness equips me with the tools to navigate them. I anchor myself in the present, grounding my awareness in the sensations of breath and body. I challenge the validity of catastrophic thoughts, reclaiming sovereignty over my mind and emotions.

Through Mindfulness, I have found not just relief from anxiety, but a profound sense of wholeness and vitality. It has given me back my life, imbuing each moment with newfound meaning and possibility.

Chapter 7

YES BUT, NO BUT...

What is Mindfulness again?

Mindfulness is the practice of paying full attention to the present moment, without judgment or distraction. It involves being aware of your thoughts, feelings, bodily sensations, and the environment around you. Mindfulness encourages you to observe these experiences without trying to change them, simply accepting them as they are.

How is Mindfulness different from meditation?

Mindfulness is a type of meditation, but it can also be practiced throughout your day in any activity. Meditation typically refers to the formal practice of sitting quietly and focusing the mind, often on the breath or a mantra. Mindfulness, on the other hand, can be practiced at any time—whether you're eating, walking, or even working—by maintaining a present-focused awareness.

What are the benefits of practicing Mindfulness?

Mindfulness offers numerous benefits, including reduced stress and anxiety, improved emotional regulation, better focus and concentration, enhanced self-awareness, and greater overall well-being. Studies have shown that Mindfulness can lead to improved mental and physical health, including better sleep, lower blood pressure, and a stronger immune system.

How do I start practicing Mindfulness?

To start practicing Mindfulness, set aside a few minutes each day to focus on your breath. Find a quiet space where you won't be disturbed. Sit comfortably, close your eyes, and focus on the sensation of your breath as it enters and leaves your body. When your mind wanders, gently bring your focus back to your breath. Over time, you can extend Mindfulness to daily activities like eating, walking, or washing dishes by staying fully present and engaged in each task.

How long should I practice Mindfulness each day?

You can start with just 5 to 10 minutes a day and gradually increase the duration as you become more comfortable with the practice. Many people find that 20 to 30 minutes of daily Mindfulness meditation is ideal for experiencing the full benefits, but even a few minutes of Mindfulness can make a difference.

Can Mindfulness help with anxiety and depression?

Yes, Mindfulness has been shown to be effective in reducing symptoms of anxiety and depression. By bringing awareness to the present moment and observing thoughts without judgment, Mindfulness can help break the cycle of negative thinking that often accompanies these conditions. Mindfulness-Based Cognitive Therapy (MBCT) is a specific approach that combines Mindfulness practices with cognitive therapy to prevent the recurrence of depression.

Is Mindfulness a religious practice?

While Mindfulness has roots in Buddhist meditation, it is a secular practice that can be embraced by people of any or no religious background. Mindfulness is simply about paying attention to the present moment and can be practiced by anyone, regardless of their beliefs.

What should I do if I find it difficult to stay focused during Mindfulness practice?

It's normal for your mind to wander during Mindfulness practice, especially when you're first starting out. When this happens, simply acknowledge that your mind has wandered and gently bring your focus back to your breath or the present moment. Over time, with regular practice, your ability to stay focused will improve.

Can I practice Mindfulness if I'm very busy?

Yes, Mindfulness is particularly valuable for busy people, as it helps you manage stress and stay focused amidst a hectic schedule. You don't need to set aside a lot of time; you can practice Mindfulness in just a few minutes each day or even while doing everyday activities like commuting, eating, or working.

What Are Some Simple Mindfulness Exercises I Can Do During the Day?

There are several easy Mindfulness exercises you can incorporate into your daily routine. Here are a few examples:

Mindful Breathing: Take a few moments to focus on your breath, noticing each inhale and exhale. This simple practice can quickly center your mind.

Body Scan: Slowly scan your body from head to toe, paying attention to any areas of tension or discomfort. Breathe into these areas, allowing them to soften and release.

Mindful Eating: Pay full attention to the experience of eating, savoring each bite. Notice the flavors, textures, and smells, being fully present with the food.

Mindful Walking: Walk slowly and deliberately, focusing on the sensation of your feet touching the ground and the movement of your body. This can bring calm and focus to everyday activities.

Mindful Listening: When conversing with someone, practice fully listening to them without planning your response or getting distracted by your own thoughts. This enhances connection and understanding.

Can Mindfulness Be Practiced in a Group?

Yes, Mindfulness can be practiced both individually and in a group setting. Group Mindfulness sessions, such as meditation classes or retreats, offer support, motivation, and a sense of community. Many people find practicing Mindfulness with others helpful, especially when starting out.

Is Mindfulness Suitable for Children?

Absolutely. Mindfulness can be highly beneficial for children, helping them develop focus, emotional regulation, and self-awareness. There are Mindfulness programs specifically designed for children, using age-appropriate exercises and activities. Practicing Mindfulness as a family can also be a wonderful way to introduce these concepts to children.

Can Mindfulness Improve My Physical Health?

Yes, Mindfulness has been linked to several physical health benefits, including lower blood pressure, reduced chronic pain, improved sleep, and a stronger immune system. By reducing stress and promoting relaxation, Mindfulness can contribute to your overall physical well-being.

How Does Mindfulness Affect the Brain?

Research has shown that regular Mindfulness practice can lead to changes in the brain. For example, it can increase the density of grey matter in areas associated with learning, memory, and emotional regulation. Mindfulness can also reduce activity in the amygdala, the brain's "fear center," which is involved in the stress response.

Can Mindfulness Help Improve Relationships?

Yes, Mindfulness can improve relationships by helping you be more present, listen actively, and respond thoughtfully instead of reacting impulsively. By cultivating Mindfulness, you can become more aware of your own emotions and needs as well as those of others, leading to more compassionate and effective communication.

What Are Common Misconceptions About Mindfulness?

One misconception is that Mindfulness is about clearing your mind. Mindfulness is not about stopping your thoughts but about observing them without attachment or judgment. Another misconception is that Mindfulness is a quick fix. While it can provide immediate benefits, it requires regular practice over time for lasting change. Lastly, Mindfulness is not only for relaxation; while it can be relaxing, its primary purpose is to cultivate awareness and presence.

Can I Measure My Progress in Mindfulness?

Progress in Mindfulness is often subtle. You may notice improvements in how you respond to stress, your ability to stay present, and your awareness of thoughts and emotions. Keeping a Mindfulness journal, where you reflect on your practice, can help track growth over time. You might also notice improvements in your overall well-being, relationships, and mental clarity.

Are There Different Types of Mindfulness Practices?

Yes, there are various types of Mindfulness practices, including:

Mindfulness Meditation: Focus on the breath, body sensations, or a specific mantra.

Loving-Kindness Meditation: Cultivate compassion and kindness towards yourself and others.

Body Scan Meditation: Bring awareness to different parts of the body in sequence, noticing any sensations or tension.

Mindful Movement: Engage in activities like yoga, Tai Chi, or walking with full attention to the body's movements.

Mindful Eating, Walking, or Listening: Bring mindful awareness to everyday activities, staying present and engaged.

Can Mindfulness Be Integrated into Other Practices, Like Dowsing?

Yes, Mindfulness can complement many practices, including Dowsing, by enhancing focus, intuition, and present-moment awareness. For instance, practicing Mindfulness before Dowsing can help clear your mind and approach the activity with greater clarity and intention. Combining Mindfulness with other practices can deepen your experience and improve outcomes.

How Do I Stay Motivated to Practice Mindfulness Regularly?

To stay motivated, start small—begin with just a few minutes a day and gradually increase the time as you become more comfortable. Consistency is key, so try to practice Mindfulness at the same time each day to build a routine. Set reminders on your phone or place sticky notes in visible areas to prompt you to practice. Joining a group can also provide support and encouragement. Finally, regularly remind yourself of the benefits you've experienced from Mindfulness, such as reduced stress or improved focus.

Chapter 8

DOWSING - BEYOND THE MAGIC WAND

After our quick look at these two fascinating practices, let's dive deeper into what they involve. By the time we get to the end of this book, we're going to be different people, with new skills and confidence. So, let's begin.

Forget the pointy hats and sparkly cloaks. Dowsing isn't some mystical practice reserved for fortune tellers and wizards. It's a surprisingly down-to-earth way to tap into our inner wisdom and connect with unseen forces. Think of it as a superpower waiting to be unleashed—a way to find hidden treasures, both literal and metaphorical, with a simple tool and a healthy dose of intuition.

Dowsing isn't magic, although it can feel that way sometimes. It's a practice of harnessing your intuition and connecting with a deeper well of information—a field some call the Universal Mind, the Akashic Record, or simply "Out There." Imagine your mind as a computer, and Dowsing as the tool that lets you tap into the vastness of the internet—the answers are all there if you know how to ask.

Who Can Dowse? You!

The good news is that practically anyone can learn to dowse. It's not about having some special gift; it's about quieting the chatter of the conscious mind and amplifying the subtle signals your intuition is already sending. While anyone can get started, mastering the art takes dedication and practice. Like any new skill, there will be bumps along the road. Don't get discouraged by early hiccups—embrace them as opportunities to learn and refine your technique.

The Dowsing Dance: Tools and Techniques

The most important Dowsing tool you have is your own mind. But to bridge the gap between your conscious awareness and the deeper information field, dowsers often use tools like pendulums, Y-rods (forked sticks), L-rods or, as mentioned earlier, something called a bobber. These tools act as amplifiers, translating the subtle movements of your hands into clear "yes" or "no" answers. It's like a conversation between your conscious mind and your subconscious, a mental dance that unveils hidden knowledge.

The source of these answers has been debated for centuries. Some believe it stems from a higher consciousness, while others see it as tapping into the collective unconscious. Regardless of the explanation, the results are undeniable. Dowsing has been used for millennia to locate water sources, minerals, and even lost objects. Most people associate Dowsing with finding water, but there's so much more to this practice.

The Many Faces of Dowsing

Dowsing isn't a one-trick pony. The British Society of Dowsers recognizes four main applications for the art—two tangible and two intangible.

The tangible applications are:

Water and Minerals: This is perhaps the most well-known use of Dowsing. With a growing global population and dwindling freshwater reserves, skilled water dowsers are becoming increasingly valuable.

Archaeology: Dowsing can be a powerful tool for archaeologists, helping them pinpoint buried ruins and artifacts with surprising accuracy. Imagine uncovering a Roman villa or an

Iron Age fort based on the subtle signals picked up by your instruments.

The intangible uses are:

Health Dowsing: This is where Dowsing gets truly fascinating—and where it becomes relevant to your Mindfulness journey. Dowsing can be used to identify imbalances in the body's energy field, helping us understand the root cause of health concerns. Some dowsers work full-time as health practitioners, not only identifying the source of mystifying illnesses but also using their skills to aid in healing.

Earth Energies: The Earth pulsates with energies that can impact our well-being. For example, underground streams can often have a negative effect on our homes or workplaces if they flow directly beneath. Dowsing can help us locate these sources of energy and identify whether they are positive or negative, allowing us to create a more harmonious environment.

Dowsing is all about connecting with our intuition, and it's a powerful tool to add to our Mindfulness toolkit, helping us connect with the unseen forces that shape our world and ourselves.

As we delve deeper into Dowsing, we'll explore the world of health Dowsing and how it can empower you on your path to Mindfulness. We'll also address the skepticism surrounding Dowsing and explore the science behind this age-old practice. So, buckle up and get ready to dowse your way to a more mindful and connected you!

The Power of Dowsing Is Limited Only by Our Imagination

When most people think of Dowsing, they imagine an elderly man striding across a field, a forked twig clutched in his hands, searching for underground water—like our earlier-mentioned friend George Applegate, who celebrated his 80th birthday by finding his 1,000th borehole. Yes, that's part of the story, but Dowsing is so much more.

It's about using simple instruments like pendulums or L-rods to answer questions, make mindful choices, and gain insights into your own well-being. It's about trusting your gut feeling, that little voice whispering guidance from within. Dowsing can unlock mysteries ranging from "Did the Universe really start with a big bang?" to "Is it going to rain today?"

Imagine this: you're standing in a supermarket, overwhelmed by a sea of salad options. Baby spinach, kale, romaine—which one is right for you today? Instead of relying on impulse or the latest fad diet, you could pull out your trusty pendulum and ask it a simple question: "Is this the best leafy green for my dinner tonight?" The pendulum might swing one way for "Yes" and another for "No," helping you navigate the nutritional jungle with a direct line to your intuition. Later, we'll delve into how to discover your "Yeses" and "Noes" when Dowsing.

Dowsing isn't about blind faith or magic spells. It's about cultivating a deeper connection with yourself and the world around you. It's about learning to trust the subtle signals your body and intuition are constantly sending. Think of it as turning up the volume on your inner GPS, guiding you towards a life filled with greater awareness and purpose.

Of course, there are skeptics who scoff at the idea of a forked stick or a weighted pendulum holding any real power. They might call it wishful thinking or a parlour trick. But here's the thing: Dowsing has been around for centuries, used by farmers, healers, and everyday people to locate water, find lost objects, check the health of animals and plants, and make informed decisions on a variety of topics. Scientists and skeptics may not be able to explain it, but the fact remains—it works.

Here's the beauty of Dowsing: you don't need a PhD in physics or a lifetime of training to give it a try. All you need is an open mind, a willingness to experiment, and a simple tool like a pendulum or a forked branch you can prune from a bush in your garden. Dowsing is a practice that anyone can learn, regardless of background or belief system.

Are you ready to ditch the concept of a magic wand and embrace the power of your own intuition? Dowsing might just be the missing piece you've been searching for on your journey to a more mindful and fulfilling life.

That's just a brief introduction to the subject of Dowsing. In the next chapter, we'll delve deeper into the world of Mindfulness, exploring how this ancient practice can be combined with Dowsing to unlock your true potential. But before we move on, remember—Dowsing isn't just about finding answers. It's about embarking on a journey of self-discovery, one swing of the pendulum, one step at a time.

Chapter 9

MINDFULNESS – A MODERN MIRACLE

Let's face it: life can often feel like a never-ending to-do list. Between work deadlines, family obligations, and the constant ping-pong of social media, it's easy to get swept away in the current, barely noticing the present moment. But what if I told you that there's a secret weapon hidden within you—a key to unlocking inner peace and navigating the chaos with a calm mind? That secret weapon, dear reader, is Mindfulness.

Now, Mindfulness might sound like new-age mumbo jumbo reserved for yogis contorted in pretzel positions, but it's far simpler than that. Mindfulness is about paying attention—on purpose—to the present moment. It's about being aware of your thoughts, feelings, and bodily sensations without judgment. It's about taking a deep breath and truly experiencing the world around you—the taste of your morning coffee, the warmth of the sun on your skin, the sound of birds chirping outside your window.

As we dive deeper into our Mindfulness journey, we'll learn how to personalize each exercise to suit our unique circumstances. Sure, group sessions have value, but Mindfulness can also be tailored to meet your individual needs. For instance, a group session might focus on breathing exercises for relaxation. However, in a personal session, you might want to address the daily stress of dealing with a bullying boss. And if you combine Mindfulness with your newfound Dowsing skills, you'll have a unique solution to a problem that's personal to you.

But let's get back to the basics: you don't need hours of meditation or a silent retreat to reap the benefits of Mindfulness. You can integrate it into your everyday life in short bursts, transforming mundane tasks into mindful moments. Washing the dishes? Instead of letting your mind wander to that overflowing inbox, focus on the sensation of the warm water on your hands and the sound of clinking plates. Taking a shower? Become aware of the spray of water, the scent of your soap, and the way your muscles relax under the warm cascade.

Even a simple five-minute Mindfulness practice can make a world of difference. It's not about achieving some zen-like state of perfect stillness. It's about becoming aware of the constant chatter in your mind and learning to gently nudge it back to the present moment. Think of it like training a playful puppy—it may wander off on tangents, but with a little patience and practice, you can guide it back to sit at your feet.

Letting Go

To be fully effective, you need to embrace the art of letting go. Not of your dreams or aspirations, but of the anxieties, worries, and negative thoughts that weigh you down. As we mentioned earlier, Mindfulness helps stop the internal chatter and creates a sense of peace. Imagine a lighter you, unburdened by the baggage of "what ifs" and "should haves." Letting go is key to unlocking a more present, joyful experience of life.

Stop Judging Yourself

That inner critic—the voice that whispers doubts and insecurities—can be a real downer. Try treating yourself with the same kindness and understanding you'd offer a friend. Would you judge a friend so harshly? It's time to extend that same grace to yourself. Yes, I mean it: be kind to you.

What's the Rush?

In our fast-paced world, slowing down feels almost revolutionary. Don't rush through life on autopilot, missing the richness of the present moment. Find joy in the simple act of being.

Pause and Breathe

Integrate short Mindfulness pauses throughout your day by taking a few conscious breaths whenever you feel stressed or overwhelmed.

The benefits of Mindfulness are vast. It can reduce stress and anxiety, improve focus and concentration, and even boost your overall well-being. It can help you break free from negative thought patterns and cultivate a sense of calm amidst the daily storm.

So, the next time you feel overwhelmed, take a deep breath and tap into the power within. Mindfulness might seem like a simple practice, but it's a powerful tool that can transform your everyday life, one mindful moment at a time. And guess what? This newfound Mindfulness will be the perfect foundation for exploring the world of Dowsing in the next chapter. After all, Dowsing requires a quiet mind and clear focus—something Mindfulness can definitely help you achieve. Together, they have what you might call a symbiotic relationship.

PART 2
Chapter 10

JOURNEY OF A THOUSAND MILES BEGINS WITH...A TOOLBOX

Now that we've peeked into the fascinating worlds of Dowsing and Mindfulness, it's time to explore in more detail the Dowsing toolbox. Just like any good explorer wouldn't venture into the wilderness empty-handed, a dowser needs a trusty tool to guide them on their journey of inner discovery. But as you know by now, the Dowsing toolkit is refreshingly simple and accessible—no high-tech gadgets or expensive equipment required. Yay!

The most iconic Dowsing tool is undoubtedly the pendulum. Imagine a simple weight—a crystal, a wedding ring, even a nut on a string—suspended from a thread or chain. This unassuming little instrument can be a powerful conduit for our intuition. Hold the string lightly between your thumb and forefinger, focus your question on the object suspended below, and watch it dance.

Now here's where a lot of people get frustrated before they've even begun. They dangle the pendulum, motionless, and ask their question. Nothing happens. They try again. Again, nothing happens. Confidence begins to ebb. They ask again, perhaps rephrasing the question in case the pendulum didn't understand the first one! Still nothing. Frustration sets in, and it's very tempting to throw the whole thing out the window and get back to familiar tasks like paying the gas bill or taking the dog for a walk. The pendulum just hangs there, mocking.

Don't despair. All you need to do is set the pendulum going in what's known as 'the search position.' With a flick of the wrist, nudge the pendulum into a diagonal swing so that it has some energy behind it. Gradually, the back-and-forth diagonal motion will transform into a uniform clockwise or anti-clockwise movement.

At this point, it's important to establish your own unique 'Yes' and 'No' signals. For many people, clockwise means 'Yes' and anti-clockwise means 'No.' But for some, it's the opposite. For others, a 'Yes' is an up-and-down motion like a head nodding, with swinging to the left and right, like a head shaking, meaning 'No.' Whatever you feel comfortable with and what works for you is your own unique response.

There is no right or wrong way, as long as the signal is consistent. A good method of checking out your Yeses and Noes is to dangle the pendulum first over your right knee and then your left—after giving it a diagonal 'nudge,' of course. As the right knee is positive and the left negative, you should get a 'Yes' movement and then a 'No.' And remember what your responses are for future reference.

There is a third reaction which you should be aware of—a confused swinging and circling that makes no sense to you. This is your pendulum's way of saying, "That's a daft question—how can I answer that correctly?" For instance, "Am I a good person?" Good in what way? Good for a laugh? Good to animals? Good for a cannibal to eat? Be specific. The Dowsing tool can't read your mind. Much like a computer, it takes things literally. Unlike you or me, it cannot judge nuances, tone of voice, or irony. It will answer you literally. When it comes to a debatable question, it won't answer at all. That is why it is so important to be precise in your questioning.

For instance, it's no good asking your pendulum, "Is there water under this field?" It will probably tell you "Yes." But while you meant "drinkable" water, it's just telling you that there's water, which turns out to be sewage. Remember: for results that are terrific, it pays to be specific! If you were a water dowser asking that last question of your forked stick, you would probably say something like, "Show me drinkable water, flowing all year round, at a rate of at least 200 liters a minute, at less than 30 meters in depth." Long-winded, yes, but your stick is left in no doubt about the answer you're seeking.

Imagine transforming from an occasional Dowsing dabbler into a highly sought-after practitioner. The key lies in mastering the art of asking specific questions.

Clarity and Focus: The Bedrock of Success

Before embarking on your Dowsing quest, ensure your mind is clear and focused. Imagine a calm lake reflecting the sky—that's the ideal state. Daily worries can cloud your intuition, so take a few deep breaths and find your center (when you are a Mindfulness covert this will come more easily to you).

Drinking enough water is also essential. Dehydration can hinder your Dowsing abilities, so stay well-hydrated throughout the day.

If you're feeling under the weather, it can also impact your results. Additionally, reversed polarity—a temporary state where your "Yes" responses register as "No" and vice versa—can occur. A simple "Thymus Thump" (three chest thumps followed by a cough) can often reverse polarity. It may sound quirky, but it works.

Persistence is key. Dowsing, like any skill, requires practice. Don't get discouraged if you don't see immediate results. Keep practicing regularly, and your confidence and accuracy will grow.

Avoid over-thinking. Excessive analysis can be a barrier. Trust your intuition and avoid fretting over the mechanics of Dowsing. Children are often natural dowsers because they approach it as a normal part of life and don't get hung up on the outcome.

Chapter 11

LET'S GET REAL

Even the most skilled dowsers experience occasional inaccuracies. Accept that there's always a margin for error (George Applegate had his failures, too).

Dowsing accuracy improves with practice—there's no shortcut to expertise. Find your Dowsing style. Experiment and discover the method that feels most comfortable and effective for you.

Don't let the 'Cosmic Joker' discourage you. There will be times when you question your abilities. This is what our friend CJ is waiting for. He knows you have what it takes to be a good dowser, and he doesn't like it. If he can make you give up, it's a win for him. Persistence is the key to overcoming these challenges.

By embracing these principles and honing your questioning skills, you'll be well on your way to becoming a confident and successful dowser. Remember, the journey is just as important as the destination. You don't become a success overnight, but stick with it, and gradually you'll transform it into a thing of wonder.

And Talking of Things of Wonder

While pendulums might steal the spotlight, let's not forget the classic L-rod. These L-shaped tools, traditionally crafted from malleable metal, have been used for centuries. The dowser holds the shorter arm of each L-rod in their hands. As they walk over an area of interest, the rods may twitch, cross, or diverge, signaling the presence of something underground. Some dowsers swear by L-rods, finding their simplicity and stability comforting.

The easiest way to make an L-rod is from a metal coat han'
Ultimately, the best Dowsing tool is the one that feels

comfortable and intuitive to you. Experiment with pendulums, L-rods, or even something unique—the key is to find an instrument that resonates with your energy.

Remember, these tools are simply extensions of your own intention and focus. Treat them with respect, cleanse them with sage smoke or running water if that resonates with you, and most importantly, trust the subtle movements they guide you towards.

But the Dowsing toolkit isn't limited to physical objects. One of the most powerful tools you possess is your own mind and body. Have you ever had a "gut feeling" about a situation? That intuitive nudge is a form of Dowsing in itself. Learn to pay attention to these subtle signals—a clenching in your stomach, a sudden warmth in your palms. Your body is an incredible biofeedback system, constantly sending you messages. By becoming more mindful and attuned to these internal whispers, you can harness the power of your intuition and gain valuable insights.

As you delve deeper into the world of Dowsing, you might encounter more unconventional tools. Some dowsers use charts or maps, while others experiment with crystals or gemstones. The possibilities are endless! The key is to approach these tools with an open mind and a sense of exploration. See what works for you, and trust your inner guide.

Map Dowsing is used extensively in Russia, particularly for military targets. The Russians are not so dismissive as the West of the counter-intuitive aspects of the practice—they just do it.

One of the most dramatic examples of map Dowsing is attributed to the legendary dowser and inventor of the world's most complex Dowsing tool, Verne Cameron (1896–1970). In 1959, during the Cold War, Cameron demonstrated his prowess by identifying the location of US and Soviet submarines using only a world map. His success led to him being banned from leaving the US by security officials! Vern later went on to invent the most versatile Dowsing instrument in the world – the Aurameter.

But to repeat, the most important tool in your Dowsing arsenal isn't something you can hold in your hand. It's the unwavering belief in your own intuition. Dowsing is a journey of self-discovery, a conversation between your conscious mind and your inner wisdom. The tools are simply there to amplify those whispers, guiding you on your path to a more mindful and empowered life.

So, grab your pendulum, your L-rod, or simply your own open mind, and get ready to embark on this exciting adventure!

Unlocking Your Hidden Superpower

We've touched on the intriguing worlds of Dowsing and Mindfulness, unpacked the toolbox of tools, and now it's time to delve into the real magic—awakening that Dowsing intuition. This isn't about acquiring some mystical power or becoming a fortune teller. It's about rediscovering a natural ability that lies dormant within us all: the ability to tap into subtle information and translate it into clear guidance. Think of it as a buried treasure waiting to be unearthed, a hidden superpower inside you waiting to be unleashed.

Now, you might be wondering, "Where exactly is this Dowsing intuition hiding, and how do I access it?" The answer lies within. Your intuition is a symphony of subtle signals—a combination of gut feelings, physical sensations, and even fleeting images or dreams. It's the voice that whispers warnings, nudges you toward opportunities, and guides you down paths aligned with your highest good. The problem? In our fast-paced world, we often drown out these whispers with the constant chatter of our minds.

The key to awakening your Dowsing intuition lies in cultivating a state of mindful awareness. Remember those Mindfulness moments mentioned earlier? Becoming present in the now, focusing on our breath, and quieting the mental noise—these practices are the foundation for unlocking your inner wisdom. The more attuned you are to your internal landscape, the easier it becomes to pick up on the subtle signals that guide your Dowsing practice.

Here's a powerful technique to jumpstart your Dowsing intuition: body Dowsing. This practice involves paying close attention to your physical sensations in response to questions or situations. Think of a simple yes-or-no question you'd like an answer to. Hold the question firmly in your mind, then focus on your body. Does your stomach clench with a feeling of "No"? Perhaps a sense of warmth in your chest signals a "Yes"? These subtle physical cues can be incredibly insightful once you learn to interpret them. There are some professional dowsers who have cast aside their Dowsing instruments in favor of just one – their bodies. I know one who just used blinking for his yes/no answers.

Another powerful tool for awakening your Dowsing intuition is visualization. Imagine yourself successfully Dowsing for something specific—a lost object, perhaps, or a hidden water source. See yourself holding your Dowsing tool, feeling confident and focused. Envision the tool responding clearly to your questions, providing answers you can trust. This practice of visualization helps prime your subconscious mind and amplify your ability to pick up on subtle cues.

Don't be discouraged if you don't experience immediate results. Like any skill, Dowsing takes practice and patience. The good news? There are countless ways to hone your intuition and build your confidence in this amazing ability. Here are some tips:

• **Start with simple questions**: Don't dive headfirst into life-altering decisions. Begin by asking your Dowsing tool yes-or-no questions about everyday matters. "Is this the right grocery store for me today?" Or "Should I wear my blue or green shirt?" These small-scale Dowsing sessions will help you build trust in your intuition and the tools you're using.

• **Keep a Dowsing journal**: Track your experiences, noting your questions, the responses you received through your Dowsing tool, and how those responses aligned with reality. Over time, you'll start to identify patterns and gain confidence in your intuition's accuracy.

• **Practice, practice, practice**: Dowsing, like any skill, improves with practice. Set aside some time each day to hone your intuition. You can use Dowsing charts (more on this specialism later) or games specifically designed to develop your Dowsing skills. The more you experiment and play, the more comfortable and confident you'll become.

• **Trust yourself**: This might be the most crucial step of all. Dowsing is a journey of self-discovery, and it hinges on trusting yourself. If a Dowsing response feels off, don't dismiss it. Explore it further, and learn to differentiate genuine intuition from wishful thinking.

Awakening your Dowsing intuition can be a transformative experience. It's about learning to trust your inner guidance, becoming more aware of the world around you, and making empowered choices aligned with your deepest desires.

So, embrace the journey, have fun experimenting, and remember, the most powerful Dowsing tool you possess is already within you. It's time to awaken your intuition and unlock the hidden superpower that has been waiting to be unleashed!

t

Chapter 12

WHAT DO I DO WHEN THE GOING GETS WEIRD?

You've embarked on your Dowsing journey, armed with your newfound knowledge and a trusty tool. You're making mindful choices, connecting with your intuition, and navigating life with a newfound sense of empowerment. But hold on a minute—what happens when your pendulum starts spinning wildly, your L-rods refuse to budge, and you keep getting silly answers?

You've encountered that character you've already been introduced to—and who all successful dowsers are familiar with—the 'Cosmic Joker.' He knows you're potentially a good dowser, so he wants to stop you in your tracks. He throws you all kinds of curveballs in the hope you'll be discouraged and give up. **Don't!** This is a battle that you will win if you're stubborn and keep on practicing. Here are some of the conditions good old CJ uses to destroy your confidence:

- **External Interference**: Electromagnetic fields, strong emotions, or even air currents can disrupt your Dowsing tool. Try Dowsing in a neutral environment, free from distractions. Ground yourself with a few deep breaths before interrogating your Dowsing instrument.

- **Ambiguous Question**: Perhaps you weren't clear enough. Instead of asking, "Is tea or coffee better for my health?" Ask, "Is tea better for my health than coffee?" Now you should get a definitive yes-or-no answer.

• **Overthinking It**: Sometimes, overanalyzing the situation can lead to a disconnect with your intuition. Relax your grip on the pendulum, take a deep breath, and allow it to respond naturally. Don't fall into the classic dowsers' trap of "paralysis by analysis."

• **Dowsing Fatigue**: Just like any physical activity, Dowsing can be tiring. Take a break, recharge your energy, and come back to your Dowsing session with a fresh focus.

• **Blocked Intuition**: Stress, emotional baggage, or negative self-talk can block your intuition. Practice Mindfulness exercises to clear your head and create space for your intuition to flow freely.

• **Nonsensical Answer**: You think you've formulated a clear question, your Dowsing tool responds definitively, but the answer seems completely illogical. That's because you haven't been specific enough. For instance, on a Wednesday, you might ask, "Is it Wednesday today?" and get a "No." But it is Wednesday today, you tell yourself. However, in some parts of the world, it might not be Wednesday. You should have phrased your question: "Is it Wednesday where I am located?" I know I bang on about this but it's crucial how you phrase your questions. You must be specific! Sermon over.

There are plenty more of these pitfalls, so be on your guard and keep plugging on despite the odd setback. The occasional Dowsing challenge shouldn't discourage you. Instead, embrace it as an opportunity to learn and grow in your skillfulness. So, keep swinging that pendulum, experimenting with your L-rods, Y-rods, or bobbers, and embrace the mysteries that unfold.

DOWSING   FOR   TRANSFORMATION: SUPERCHARGING YOUR LIFE

Dowsing isn't just about finding lost keys or hidden water sources. It's a powerful tool for transformation—a way to tap into your inner wisdom and supercharge your life on multiple levels. We've explored the foundations of Dowsing and Mindfulness, conquered challenges, and now it's time to delve into the transformative potential of this practice. Get ready to explore environmental Dowsing, personal healing, emotional awareness, and even your connection to the greater good—all through the lens of Dowsing.

Our environment has a profound impact on our well-being. Dowsing can be a powerful tool for creating a harmonious and supportive living space. Here are some ways to use Dowsing to transform your environment:

Identifying Negative Energy Pockets:

Does a particular corner of your home feel stagnant or draining? Use your Dowsing tool (I prefer an L-rod here) to identify areas with negative energy flow. You probably need only one rod. Hold it steady with the nose slightly down so gravity keeps it balanced, and ask it to point you to the nearest negative energy spiral. Then start walking slowly forward. Your rod should swing in a particular direction. Follow that direction; it might veer again, so keep following, down the corridor or into another room until it swings dramatically, as if crossing with its invisible partner. You have found your negative energy spiral.

Once identified, you can employ techniques like smudging or placing crystals to cleanse the space and restore positive energy. Or, using your intent, you can simply command the energies to transmute into beneficial energy. I say something like, "I remove all detrimental energies here and bless this room with beneficial energy to bring balance, harmony, health, and healing to the complete being—physical, emotional, mental, and spiritual—of all who enter here." Then I usually dowse again, asking, "Show me the nearest detrimental energy spiral." If your Dowsing tool refuses to move, it means there isn't any. Job done.

Optimizing Furniture Placement:

Furniture arrangement can significantly impact the energy flow in your home. Use Dowsing to determine the most optimal placements for furniture pieces, promoting a sense of balance and harmony within your living space. Just like searching for detrimental energies, we can wield our rods or pendulum to locate the best places. Say something like, "All things considered for the well-being of me and my family, where would be the best place to locate the settee?" Use the same wording in all rooms for beds (very important as you don't want to be sleeping over a negative energy line), chairs, desks, the dining table, etc. If you prefer to use a pendulum to locate these optimum spaces, swing it into the search mode, ask your question, and then wait until it steadies itself in a certain direction. Slowly follow that direction until it switches to your version of "Yes."

Chapter 13

WHO AM I? DOWSING YOUR WAY TO SELF-DISCOVERY

Dowsing isn't a magic bullet for curing diseases, but it can be a powerful tool for promoting self-healing and overall well-being. Here are some ways to use Dowsing for personal transformation:

Identifying Food Sensitivities:

Do you suspect certain foods might be causing digestive issues or fatigue? Dowsing can help you pinpoint potential food sensitivities, allowing you to make informed dietary choices that promote gut health and overall well-being. Draw up, or get hold of, a list of food allergies or intolerances like milk, wheat, eggs, shellfish, peanuts, and so on. Put the list on a flat surface in front of you, get into your Dowsing zone, and ask your pendulum, "Show me any of the following substances to which I have an allergy or intolerance." Set your pendulum swinging into search mode and slowly run your finger down the list. When you get to a suspect substance, your pendulum will swing into your "Yes" movement. Make a mental note and move on until you have completed the list. Say you have identified five intolerances; dowse these one by one, asking, "On a scale of one to 10, with 10 being the highest, how serious is this food (say shellfish) as a threat to my gut health?" Swinging into search mode again, say, "Is it more than five?" If the answer is "Yes," go on to six, seven, and so on until you get another "Yes." If your first answer was less than five, use the same principle to dowse the numbers below five. At the end of the exercise, you will know which foods to avoid at all costs and which you might indulge in very occasionally.

Chakra Balancing:

Chakras are energy centers within the body. Dowsing can be used to identify imbalances in your chakras, prompting you to explore healing techniques like meditation, yoga, or crystals to restore balance and enhance energy flow. Again, using a pendulum, you can ask it of each chakra, "Does my Crown Chakra need re-balancing?" "My Brow Chakra?" and so on, all the way to the Root Chakra. You will now know which of your energy centers need attention. The method you use to restore balance is your individual choice, but, in the end, you are using your intent. If you want to continue using your pendulum, you can. Swinging it into its positive mode, point the index finger of your free hand to whichever chakra needs attention and say something like, "I bless my (Crown Chakra, for instance) with balance and harmony, health and healing, enabling it to work with 100% effectiveness with all my other chakras." Wait until the pendulum has finished its twirling and then say similar words to all chakras that need attention.

Crystal Selection:

Crystals are believed to possess unique healing properties. Dowsing can help you select crystals that resonate with your specific needs, promoting emotional well-being, physical vitality, or spiritual growth. I use either a pendulum or rod for this. After setting the task in my head, such as, "Show me the best crystal to inspire and guide my life in the future to its highest purpose," I would ask my rod to point me to the best one for me, or I might swing my pendulum into search mode and point at each crystal in turn. When the swing "goes positive," that's your special crystal.

Dowsing emotions:

Our emotions are powerful forces that shape our lives. Dowsing can be a valuable tool for understanding and managing our emotional landscape. For instance, if we're feeling stuck in a cycle of anger, anxiety, or sadness, Dowsing can help us identify the root cause. "Why am I feeling this way? Is it something deep in my psyche? No. Is it caused by events over the last few days? Yes. Is it to do with a relationship? Yes. With someone close to me? Is it a work colleague? Yes." As you narrow down the search, answers will float into your head. You'll be thinking, "It was that argument I had with my boss. I thought I'd put it out of my mind, but now I realize it's something I've got to deal with." So your pendulum has empowered you to address the problem at its source, helping your emotional balance.

Finding Emotional Release Techniques:

Having identified the problem, you can dowse for the best way to restore your equilibrium before tackling your boss. So ask your pendulum for the best balm for your soul at this moment. Dowse options like journaling, spending time in nature, or perhaps meditation might be just what you need. Your trusty pendulum will guide you. Sometimes, the most important emotional message lies beneath the surface. Dowsing can help you connect with your inner wisdom, providing guidance on navigating emotional challenges and promoting emotional well-being.

Dowsing the environment:

Feeling passionate about environmental issues? Dowsing can be used to identify areas in need of environmental restoration or to explore sustainable solutions for your community. Here's where you have to think through the environmental challenges facing your locality and then, once you have a list, dowse the order of priority. You know how to do it by now. But remember, be specific. Not, "Does the local park need cleaning up?" but rather, "Should I organize a litter pick this weekend at our local park?"

Plugging into the collective unconscious:

The world is a complex web of interconnected energy. Dowsing can be used to tap into the collective consciousness, offering insights into global challenges and ways to contribute to positive change. This may sound like a rather tall order, but even one person can make a positive difference. You could dowse, "Is social media inflaming hatred and despair in the world?" Yes. You can then resolve that from this moment, any contribution you make to Facebook, Twitter/X, or Instagram will be positive and wholesome.

Finding Geopathic Stress Zones:

Geopathic stress (more on this important topic later) refers to disturbances in the Earth's energy field. These zones can disrupt sleep patterns and overall well-being (see my comment above on finding the best place for your bed). Dowsing can help you identify these areas in your home, allowing you to take steps to mitigate their effects (as per Negative Energy Pockets above).

Beyond the Techniques:

Dowsing for transformation is more than just a collection of techniques. It's a philosophy, a way of approaching life with an open mind and a willingness to tap into the unseen forces that shape our reality. Here are some additional tips to embrace this transformative journey:

Intention is Key:

Dowsing is a collaborative effort between your conscious mind and your intuition. Approach each session with a clear intention, focusing your thoughts on the question you seek to answer.

Trust Your Gut:

Dowsing isn't about achieving absolute certainty. Learn to trust your gut feeling, even if the Dowsing response seems unexpected. Sometimes, the most profound insights lie beyond the realm of logic.

Maintain a Beginner's Mind:

The journey of Dowsing is a lifelong exploration. Approach your practice with a sense of curiosity and openness, always seeking to learn and grow as a dowser.

Chapter 14

I'VE TRIED AND TRIED, BUT IT'S JUST NOT WORKING

Those who often end up being the best dowsers sometimes suffer a discouraging start. No matter how hard they try, somehow the answers come out wrong. This is our friend the Cosmic Joker at work. He spots good dowsers and does everything to discourage them. Don't despair, here's a reminder of some practical tips:

Relaxation:

Dowsing requires a relaxed state of mind. If you're feeling tense or stressed, take a few deep breaths and try again when you feel calmer.

Focus:

Maintain a clear mental image of what you're searching for. The clearer the picture, the easier it is for your intuition to guide the Dowsing tool.

Hydration:

Dehydration can hinder Dowsing. Make sure you're drinking plenty of water throughout the day.

Practice:

Just like any skill, Dowsing takes practice. Don't get discouraged if you don't see results immediately. Keep practicing regularly, and you'll gradually improve your ability to connect with your intuition.

Remember, some people experience success with Dowsing right away, while others take more time. Be patient with yourself and enjoy the process of learning and developing your unique skill.

Chapter 15

CHARTING YOUR WAY TO DEEPER INSIGHTS

Going Beyond Yes or No:

As your Dowsing practice evolves, you'll likely crave more nuanced answers than simple "Yes" or "No." When seeking specifics—like someone's health status, ideal garden plants, or the type of Geopathic Stress affecting a location—Dowsing charts become your secret weapon.

So What Are These Dowsing charts?

They are diagrams divided into sections representing percentages, probabilities, health gauges, the alphabet, and more. Dowsing chart books offer a vast array of options for virtually any topic. For instance, Dale Olson's book of charts includes:

- Vitamins / Essential & Trace Minerals / Amino Acids
- Food Supplements
- Enzymes for Digestion
- Nutrition & Food Allergies / Adverse Effects
- Herbal Remedies
- Flower Essence Remedies

- Systems of the Body / Glandular (Endocrine) System
- Source of Condition / Origin of Dis-ease / Dysfunction

- Healing Remedies
- Relationship Compatibility
- Personal Motivators

- Who is Involved – Their Relationship to You
- How to Change My Life
- Chakras
- Gemstones
- Directions / Degrees / Distance
- House Inventory
- Soil Chart
- Business Decision Analysis

How Do They Work?

With your pendulum or rod in the standard search position (diagonally swinging), ask your specific question. For example, using the percentage chart, ask, "What's the chance of rain today?" The pendulum will settle over a section, revealing the percentage likelihood.

Don't feel pressured to buy charts. You can create your own as you gain experience or delve deeper into a particular area. If you haven't yet got that kind of confidence, Juanita Ott's website (mirrorwaters.com) offers downloadable starter charts to get you going.

For those new to Dowsing, another free resource is Walt Woods' renowned publication, "Letter to Robin: A Mini Course in Pendulum Dowsing" (lettertorobin.org), which provides a downloadable general chart—a perfect springboard for your Dowsing journey.

For those drawn to the psychic realm, Dowsing charts become an invaluable tool, offering a deeper understanding and empowering you to navigate life's complexities.

Congratulations!

You've now embarked on the fascinating journey of Dowsing, awakening your intuition, and navigating life with a newfound sense of empowerment. But the Dowsing adventure doesn't stop here. There's a whole world waiting to be explored, filled with advanced techniques, supportive communities, and opportunities to deepen your practice.

As your confidence grows, you'll naturally seek to extend the range of your Dowsing. This section delves into the intricate mechanics of this and the techniques that will make it effective. As we journey together, we'll sometimes stray from the conventional—like finding water, minerals, and archaeological sites—to explore its more esoteric facets, such as healing and subtle energies.

Along the way, keep an eye out for opportunities to apply what you've learned and improve your techniques by integrating a Mindfulness approach. For instance, consider how Mindfulness might enhance your focus or how psychic applications of Dowsing—channeling information from other dimensions, for instance—might be enhanced by being in a Mindfulness zone.

IF YOU'RE GOING NO-WHERE YOU'LL NEED A MAP!

Beyond the familiar realms of Dowsing lie fascinating yet unusual applications—map Dowsing and remote healing, for example. Imagine pinpointing a lost object across continents or sending healing energies to a loved one from afar. Let's delve for a moment into these extraordinary practices and explore the potential connection to the enigmatic world of quantum mechanics.

Map Dowsing: A Psychic GPS

We've already been introduced to Map Dowsing through the extraordinary feats of Verne Cameron. Now let's look at the topic in a bit more detail. Map Dowsing utilizes a pendulum to locate places, people, or objects anywhere on the globe. Unlike traditional Dowsing, which interacts directly with physical objects, map Dowsing transcends physical limitations. While the exact science behind map Dowsing remains elusive, some theories suggest it taps into an invisible "information field," where the map acts as a focus for the dowser's intent—something like how a medium might use a crystal ball in a psychic reading.

Or perhaps the map interacts with subtle magnetic fields or energetic signatures linked to the target location. The truth is we humans love to have an explanation for everything, including those phenomena that defy explanation. Map Dowsing is one of those phenomena. How can anyone dangle a pendulum over a printed representation of a town, say, and locate a lost pet? But it happens. Or pinpoint the likely location of oil under the sands of a Middle Eastern country? The celebrated psychic Uri Geller didn't earn his fortune from TV appearances but by Dowsing for oil, sometimes using maps. I've told the following story in a previous book, but it bears repeating as it provides dramatic proof of Dowsing's seemingly magical (or even mystical) powers:

In 1991, when her daughter's rare, hand-carved harp was stolen, Associate Professor Elizabeth Lloyd Mayer, clinical supervisor at the University of California, Berkeley's Psychology Clinic, did something extraordinary for a dyed-in-the-wool scientific thinker. After the police failed to turn up any leads, a friend suggested she call a dowser, who specialized in finding lost objects. With nothing to lose—and almost as a joke—Dr. Mayer agreed. Within two days, and without leaving his Arkansas home 1500 miles away, the dowser located the exact California street coordinates where the harp was found. What followed turned Dr.

Mayer's familiar world of science and rational thinking upside down.

Deeply shaken, yet driven to understand what had happened, Mayer began a fourteen-year journey of discovery that ended in her writing her bestseller *Extraordinary Knowing*, which explores what science has to say about this episode and countless other "inexplicable" phenomena. From Sigmund Freud's writings on telepathy to secret CIA experiments on remote viewing, from leading-edge neuroscience to the strange world of quantum physics, Dr. Mayer researched a wealth of credible and fascinating information about the psychic world where the mind seems to trump the laws of nature.

This book you are holding now goes one step further—it will make you part of this world, and this world will become part of you.

Chapter 16

I'M JUST A BEGINNER, DON'T I NEED MORE EXPERIENCE TO MAP DOWSE?

This is one of the wonders of Dowsing, you don't have to be a grizzled veteran. If you are determined enough you can. There are various approaches, and here are two popular ones:

Grid Technique:

With a map containing the target in front of you, after focusing your mind and clearly visualizing it, slowly slide a ruler or something with a straight edge from left to right across the map or sketch, asking your Dowsing tool to indicate when the leading edge of the ruler hits whatever it is you are seeking. Then draw a line with a pencil from top to bottom of the map.

Next, repeat the exercise, this time moving the straight edge from top to bottom of the search area, again asking your Dowsing device to tell you when you have reached the target. Where the two lines cross is your location. A variation of this method is to run the ruler from opposite corners.

Pendulum Technique:

Another technique is to ask your pendulum to swing towards the target and follow this direction until the swing changes to a circular movement. One dowser I know made himself a miniature L-rod, which points at the location as he moves it around the periphery of the map. When it locks onto a definite direction, he slowly follows the line until the rod swings to one side.

Just like any other Dowsing technique, a calm and focused mind is crucial for success in map Dowsing. Mindfulness practices like meditation can help you achieve this state. By quieting your inner chatter and focusing your intention, you enhance the accuracy of your Dowsing "readings."

REMOTE HEALING: CONNECTING ACROSS SPACE AND TIME

Many dowsers possess a natural affinity for healing, extending their abilities to something called remote healing. The core principle lies in the belief that time and space are not barriers when connecting through energy. Proponents of remote healing suggest that dis-ease arises from disruptions in the human energy field. The healer's intent, like a beacon, targets this disruption, reconnecting the person's energy with a universal source of well-being, often referred to as the "Universal Matrix."

You can try this using your pendulum. Say you have a friend living 3,000 miles away, and they've emailed you to ask if you can ease the pain in their arthritic hands. Visualize your friend, homing in on their wrists, and set your pendulum to swing in its 'No' (negative) position. As it swings, imagine you are drawing out the pain from the joints. Allow the swing to continue as long as it wants. This could be anything from 30 seconds to 10 minutes. Once it has stopped, it has 'sucked' the discomfort out. Then imagine sending those black energies to the light where they will be dealt with in accordance with Divine will.

Next, start your pendulum circling in its 'Yes' (positive) mode, and imagine healing energies filling all the spaces left by the removal of the pain. While the pendulum is moving, mentally keep those vibrations burrowing into the joint. When the twirling finally stops, your job is done. At this point—and this is very important—have supreme confidence that the healing has happened and then forget it. Allow the Universe to do its work. If you keep wondering or want to email your friend to ask how they are, it's like picking at a scab. Put the whole episode from your mind and get on with your normal routine. The healing has happened. Believe.

DOWSING AS A DIAGNOSTIC TOOL

Interestingly, some healers use Dowsing tools to diagnose the root cause of an ailment, often believed to be emotional. They will likely use a chart and allow their pendulum to indicate the source of the problem. Then they'll use the technique, like the one above, to tackle it. However, some prefer a more sophisticated instrument, but which still has Dowsing at the heart of the process. In popular parlance, they are employing the magic of the "black box," and the practice is known as **Radionics.**

Radionics is a fascinating methodology that bridges the gap between Dowsing and remote healing. It utilizes specialized Dowsing instruments to "tune in" to a person's energy field, even if they're miles away. Similar to map Dowsing, a witness (like a hair sample) can act as a surrogate for the person receiving the healing.

According to the **Radionics Association**, it is a method of sending precisely defined healing energy to people, animals, or plants, no matter where they are in the world. This is exactly the same principle as 'distant' or 'remote' healing or Dowsing. It's worth quoting in full the Radionics Association's official definition:

"The name reflects the view of early practitioners that they were 'broadcasting' healing, but we now believe that radionic treatment occurs at a level of reality where there is no distance between us. This is a challenging concept, but it is entirely compatible with modern physics and also with the ancient mystic teaching that at some level we are all one, and that at this level exchanges of healing energy can occur."

The RA goes on:

"Fundamental to radionics is the view that a living body has a subtle energy field which sustains and vitalizes it. If the field is weakened, for example by stress or pollution, then eventually the physical body also becomes weak, leaving it susceptible to illness. The aim of radionics is to identify the weaknesses in this field and to correct them, and thereby alleviate or prevent physical or emotional dis-ease. This subtle field cannot be accessed using our conventional senses. Radionic practitioners use a specialized Dowsing technique to both identify the sources of weakness in the field and to select specific treatments to overcome them."

QUANTUM ENTANGLEMENT: A SCIENTIFIC LINK?

The concept of remote healing aligns with the scientific theory of **Quantum Entanglement**. This theory suggests that subatomic particles, the building blocks of everything, are interconnected. Perhaps this inherent connection allows for distant healing to occur.

EXPLORING THE POTENTIAL: A RESPONSIBLE APPROACH

While map Dowsing and remote healing present intriguing possibilities, it's important to maintain a balanced perspective. These practices should not replace conventional medical care. However, they can be valuable tools for promoting well-being when used responsibly and in conjunction with traditional treatments.

Chapter 17

THE JOURNEY CONTINUES

As you delve deeper into the world of Dowsing, remember that the journey is just as important as the destination. Embrace the process of learning, experiment with different techniques, and cultivate a sense of wonder as you explore these fascinating, and often unconventional, applications of Dowsing. Keep an open mind, trust in your intuition, and always be willing to expand your knowledge. The path of Dowsing offers endless possibilities for personal transformation, environmental harmony, and connection to the larger energies of the universe. So take your pendulum, your rod, and your intent—and let the journey continue.

Dowsing Goes Woo-Woo – But Its Results Are True True

Dowsing, the art of using pendulums or rods to tap into hidden knowledge, offers a powerful path for self-discovery and informed decision-making. However, the true potential of Dowsing lies in venturing beyond the limitations of pre-defined questions and charts by establishing a connection with your inner guide and exploring the vast realms of intuition and spirit.

The Spirit Guide: Your Interdimensional Ally

For those who believe in matters of the spirit, Dowsing becomes a powerful tool for communication. Imagine your spirit guide as a wise entity residing in another dimension, offering guidance and protection. While some may have encountered their spirit guide spontaneously, Dowsing provides a structured approach to initiate this connection.

Before embarking on this journey, quiet your mind (Mindfulness helps). Find a peaceful space, free from distractions.

Sit comfortably, take a few deep breaths, and allow your thoughts to settle. Imagine yourself walking along a sun-dappled path through a field teeming with vibrant butterflies. As you walk, inhale the calming scent of grass and feel a gentle summer breeze caress your skin.

The path leads you to a friendly woodland. The trees seem to radiate a sense of safety. Sunlight filters through the canopy, casting shifting shadows on the forest floor. As you continue, wildlife scurries around you—rabbits nibbling, squirrels scampering, and a fox momentarily crossing your path. Everything speaks of harmony; a perfect balance of nature.

In the distance, you glimpse a shaft of sunlight illuminating a clearing. Nestled there sits a small, crooked cottage. The path leads directly to its ajar front door. Gently pushing it open, you step inside and walk down a short passage to another door. You gently push it open and see a figure.

Meeting Your Guide

It is shrouded in the sun's rays, making it impossible to discern their gender. To your surprise, you feel no fear or apprehension. A chair sits opposite the figure, and an irresistible urge compels you to sit down. As you approach, you realize this is your spirit guide. Seated, you see their face, and a voice gently speaks your name.

Now, you are free to ask any questions: their name, how long they've known you (past lifetimes included), their role in your life, and their preferred communication methods (clairvoyance, clairaudience, telepathic dialogue, or Dowsing).

Gratitude and Integration

Once the conversation concludes, express your gratitude and retrace your steps. Mentally count backwards from five to zero, and open your eyes. On returning to this world, meticulously write down everything you remember. These details may fade with time, so documentation is crucial. From now on, begin each Dowsing session by mentally greeting your guide and seeking their assistance with your project. Ultimately, they determine what information to reveal.

What About Your Guardian Angel?

While similar, spirit guides and guardian angels are distinct entities. Guardian angels, immortal messengers, act as intermediaries between God and humanity. Everyone has a personal guardian angel, and countless others are available—you just have to ask! How to connect? Thousands of online rituals exist, but the key aspects remain the same: set aside time in a quiet place and maintain a spirit of faith and trust.

Dowsing provides a head start as it naturally induces an alpha brainwave state conducive to spiritual connection. Begin by asking your pendulum if establishing contact with your guardian angel is possible at this moment. A positive response signifies you can proceed.

While whirling your pendulum in a 'Yes' motion, ask for a message. Relax your mind and wait for a response, which could be clairaudient (a voice), a mental image, or a feeling of knowing. Trust your intuition and acknowledge any message received. Express your gratitude and convey your desire for a lasting connection. The more you practice, the more communication will deepen.

When Your Dowsing Rods Become Your Time Machine

Yes, our Dowsing rods can take us on a trip through time (sort of)! Dowsing won't send us hurtling through centuries, but it can help us unlock the past and even peek a little into the future. Here's how:

Uncovering History's Secrets

Imagine discovering how old a monument is just by using your pendulum! Dowsing helps gauge the age of something by picking up on its energetic signature. This is how archaeologists, using Dowsing, can build a detailed picture of ancient sites—their purpose, construction methods, and even past events. For instance, if you wanted to know the age of an ancient wall in your village whose history has been lost in the mists of time, put one hand on the wall and ask your pendulum, "Is this wall over 1,000 years old?" Set it in the search position, and if it says "No," ask, "Over 500?" If it's a Yes, ask "Over 600?" No. "Over 550?" Yes. "560?" Yes. "570?" No. So, you know the wall was built between 560 and 570 years ago. You can further refine your search by Dowsing each year between the two numbers.

The Remanence Effect

This is where things get mind-blowing (if your mind hasn't been blown already). Dowsing can tap into the lingering energy traces of objects or people long gone. Think of it like following a faint footprint. Imagine a dowser tracing the outline of a demolished church, complete with its layout! Or Dowsing the remains in a grave and finding out about the life it once lived.

Future Forecasts (with Limits)

Dowsing can offer glimpses into the future, but with a big caveat—it can't be used for personal gain. Wondering if you'll get that dream job interview? Go for it! But forget about trying to Dowse the lottery numbers. Dowsing is all about ethical use, so keep it focused on genuine needs. In fact, unethical dowsers who have deliberately used their skills to secure a personal advantage at the expense of someone else find their plans go badly awry and they lose their divining power.

Chapter 18

KEEP THESE THINGS IN MIND

Experience matters

Especially when dealing with remanence, experience helps avoid getting misled by residual energies. For instance, you might Dowse for your lost keys, only to be led to their usual spot, which you find is empty. That's remanence at play—you were picking up the invisible energies left by the keys from repeatedly depositing them in the same place.

Ask Specific Questions

Clear questions are key! (Sorry about the pun.) Instead of a broad "Where are my keys?" ask, "Where are my daughter's missing car keys NOW?" This rules out any confusion and ensures you're picking up on the correct energy signature.

Chatting with Your Furry (or Feathered) Friend

Forget Dr. Doolittle—you won't be having full conversations with your pet anytime soon. But with Dowsing, you can develop a mind-to-mind connection and gain valuable insights into their world.

Here's How It Works

1. **Make a Connection**: Start by gently placing one hand on your pet. This creates an energetic link between you. Use your other hand for your Dowsing tool—a pendulum works well.

2. **Ask Specific Questions**: The key to success is clear, concise questions. Emotions cloud things, so try to approach it neutrally. Think, "I'm open to whatever the answer is."

3. **Get to the Root of the Problem**: Let's say your dog, Daisy, has a sore leg. Is it arthritis, a sprain, or something else? Use your

pendulum to ask a series of Yes-or-No questions to narrow it down. For example: "Is Daisy's limp caused by a physical problem?" Then eliminate possibilities: "Skeletal damage?" "Muscular?" Keep going until you find the culprit.

4. **Talk it Out with Daisy (optional)**: Once you have some answers, you can talk directly to Daisy (even if she doesn't talk back!). For example, "Did you catch your paw in some bushes?" The swing of your pendulum will give you the answer.

5. **Take Action**: Based on what you learn, you can make informed decisions. Is it a minor injury that will heal on its own? Or is a trip to the vet necessary?

By regularly Dowsing with your pet, you'll deepen your understanding and build a stronger bond. You might even save some money if Dowsing reveals a simple issue that can be handled at home. So, grab your Dowsing tool and start talking to your furry (or feathered) friend!

Oh, and don't forget your plants!

Just like animals, plants might not chat back, but that doesn't mean they lack a form of intelligence you can connect with. Remember Cleve Backster, the lie-detector expert? Back in the day, he did some fascinating experiments that suggested plants respond to our thoughts and emotions! A quick reminder of Cleve's story:

Plants as Mind Readers?

Backster hooked a polygraph (a lie-detector) up to a plant and noticed a reaction when he thought about harming it. He even found similar responses from things like cut leaves and yogurt! This research opened doors to a new way of thinking about communication with living things.

You don't need fancy equipment to chat with your greenery. A simple pendulum will do. Here's how:

1. **Plant Placement**: Gently touch your plant and ask if it's happy in its current spot. Your Dowsing instrument will give you a Yes or No. If the answer's No, the pendulum can help guide you to a better location. It might swing back and forth and point in a specific direction. However, your rods might be handier. Use one and ask it to take you to the ideal spot where your plant will flourish. Move your hand forward, and this motion will give the rod some energy, and it will swing in a certain direction. Move forward, following its lead, until it swings as if crossing with its invisible partner. You've found the ideal location.

2. **Plant Health Check**: Is your plant looking a little off? Dowsing can help diagnose the problem. Ask questions like, "Do you need more water?" or "Is there too much shade?" By focusing and keeping an open mind, you can get the answers you need to help your plant thrive.

By regularly Dowsing and communicating with your plants, you can create a flourishing garden and a deeper connection with the natural world around you.

Stonehenge – What a Story It Had to Tell

Have you ever felt a strange pull toward a particular rock or crystal? Maybe there's more to it than meets the eye! According to some theories, everything, even tiny atoms, might have a kind of intelligence. Dowsing allows us to tap into this and potentially communicate with stones, especially at powerful, ancient sacred sites.

Embark on Your Own Dowsing Dialogue with the Stones

1. **Quiet the Chatter**: Logic takes a backseat here. Relax your mind and open yourself to the possibility of connection.

2. **Tune In**: Focus on the energy of the stones and let it mingle with yours. Notice any emotions or feelings that arise—don't overthink them, just acknowledge them.

3. **Ask Your Questions**: As you explore the site, feel free to ask anything that piques your curiosity. Here are some examples to get you started:

- When were these stones placed here?
- What purpose did they serve?
- Do they still hold power?
- Are there hidden water sources or energy lines nearby?
- Can we connect with other sacred sites?
- Can the stones offer guidance or healing?
- Is there a special spot I should stand in?

Remember:

- Always show respect by asking permission from the spirit of the place before entering.
- Take steps to protect yourself energetically before starting your Dowsing dialogue.

Dowsing standing stones can be a profound experience, fostering a deeper connection to the natural world and unlocking the wisdom of these ancient giants.

YOU MAY NOT, BUT YOUR BODY WILL (ALWAYS TELL THE TRUTH, THAT IS)

The Power of Muscle Testing

Have you ever wished you could get clear answers to life's challenges? Look beyond the pendulum! Muscle testing, also known as Applied Kinesiology, offers a fascinating way to tap into your body's wisdom and gain valuable insights.

How Does It Work?

Muscle testing is based on the idea that strong muscles indicate "Yes" or "true," while weak muscles indicate "No" or "false." Here's a simple exercise to try with a partner:

1. **Partner Up**: Find a willing participant.

2. **Get in Position**: Ask your partner to stand with their arm outstretched and relaxed.

3. **Light Touch**: Place two fingers on their arm just above the wrist.

4. **The Test**: Have them state a true statement, like their own name. Gently push down on their arm. If the arm resists easily, it's a "strong" response (true).

5. **Falsehood Check**: Now, have them say a false statement, like a different name. This time, the arm should feel weaker to push down (false).

You can now interrogate your partner on all manner of topics. The human body seems to have an almost magical talent for getting at the truth.

Beyond Yes or No

Muscle testing can go beyond simple true/false questions. With practice, you can use it to:

• **Find Hidden Negativity**: Is there something draining your energy in your environment? Muscle testing can help pinpoint it.

• **Make Choices with Confidence**: Feeling stuck between job offers? Muscle testing can offer guidance on which path might be a better fit.

• **Uncover Food Sensitivities**: Wondering if a particular food is causing you problems? Muscle testing can provide clues.

Important Considerations

• **Openness is Key**: Both you and your partner need to be open to the process for it to work effectively.

• **Practice Makes Perfect**: The more you practice muscle testing, the more comfortable and accurate you'll become.

• **Focus on the Now**: Muscle testing is generally best for questions about the present or immediate future.

Muscle testing is a powerful tool for self-discovery and decision-making. While it may seem unusual, it can be a valuable addition to your intuitive toolkit. Please note: muscle testing is not a replacement for professional medical advice. Always consult with a healthcare professional for any health concerns.

Chapter 19

DON'T BRING YOUR TROUBLES HOME – IT MAY HAVE ENOUGH ALREADY!

Ever felt inexplicably drained in a particular room or woken up unrefreshed despite a full night's sleep? These could be signs of something called Geopathic Stress (GS), a term used to describe harmful earth energies that can disrupt our well-being.

GS encompasses various natural and man-made phenomena believed to create negative energy fields like:

- Underground water streams
- Geological faults
- Certain mineral concentrations
- Electromagnetic fields from power lines and electronics
- Psychic manifestations (according to some)

These energies can intersect and create concentrated zones that interact with our body's energies.

How Can Dowsing Help?

While scientific instruments might not be sensitive enough to detect GS, Dowsing can. Once you've had enough practice and are confident with your Dowsing tool, you can ascertain if there are any detrimental emanations in your home or workplace and locate them. The good news is that Dowsing can also be used to neutralize GS! Here's a run-through:

1. **Locate the Source**: Using your Dowsing tool, pinpoint the areas with negative energy. Enter a relaxed state and visualize these energies transforming from detrimental into beneficial. This

happens through the power of the human mind, which I explore in great detail in my other books. If you prefer to call on an outside source, you can ask your spirit guides or higher power for assistance.

2. **Confirm the Shift**: Once finished, dowse again to confirm that the negative energy has been neutralized. Your tool should tell you that not only is the negative gone, but it's been replaced by positive vibrations.

Long-Term Maintenance

While Dowsing offers a powerful solution, it's important to remember that new negative energies are always being created (if you or your partner have had a bad day, these feelings infect your surroundings). Here's how to maintain a positive environment:

• **Mind Over Matter**: Negative thoughts and emotions can contribute to harmful energy, so practice positive thinking and cultivate a harmonious atmosphere in your home.

• **Be Aware of External Influences**: Limit exposure to harmful electromagnetic fields from electronics whenever possible.

The Power Within

Dowsing is a reminder that we have more influence over our environment than we might think. By harnessing our intuition and intention, we can create a healthy and balanced space for ourselves and our loved ones.

When Dowsing Gets Spooky

Dowsing isn't just about finding water! As you know, everything is energy, and Dowsing can help us tap into unseen realms. But this invisible world can be a mixed bag, so let's enter the Twilight Zone and talk about energies normally outside our visible spectrum—like spirit attachments—and how to protect ourselves.

Invisible Neighbors?

Imagine our world as a bustling marketplace. We see the physical objects, the people, the stuff they're selling—things we can touch. We're part of this marketplace and play our part in it. But there's also an unseen realm, teeming with energy of all kinds, including spirits of once-living beings, as well as intelligences that have never had an earthly incarnation. Sometimes, these spirits might hitch a ride on our energy field, feeding off our vitality and running our batteries down.

How Do They Get There?

These attachments can latch onto us when we're feeling vulnerable—stressed, sad, or just worn out. Think of it like having a leaky aura. Just like moths to a flame, these spirits are drawn to that low energy.

Spotting the Signs

So how do you know if you have an unwelcome guest? Here are some red flags:

- Feeling drained and sluggish
- Mood swings and irritability
- Difficulty concentrating
- Unexplained aches and pains
- Feeling like you're not yourself

The good news is, you're not powerless! Here's how to politely show your spectral guest the door:

Shine a Light: Visualize a brilliant white light surrounding you, a protective bubble that keeps out negativity. Imagine it pushing outward, cleansing your aura.

Set Boundaries

Talk to the spirit calmly and firmly. Tell them they're not welcome and to move on to the light. You can even use your Dowsing tool to help guide them. Twirl your pendulum in an anti-clockwise motion (if that's your No direction—if your No is clockwise, use that motion). As the weight circles, think or say, "I am removing all detrimental energy from my aura and my being." Then imagine the movement winding the attachment out of your energy field. Once the pendulum slows down, switch direction into a Yes mode. Keep it going as you say, "I am now replacing all the spaces left with beneficial energy, bringing balance, harmony, health, and healing to my complete being—physical, emotional, mental, and spiritual. In love and gratitude, Amen."

If you feel uncertain that your unwanted intruder has actually left (some can be stubborn), ask for help from a higher power, such as angels or spirit guides, to escort the spirit away.

Staying Positive

The best defense against these sneaky stalkers is staying positive, confident, and connected to your inner light. In this way, you'll naturally repel negativity. Dowsing is a great tool to help you stay balanced and protected. Create a ritual for yourself in which you and your divining tool regularly perform a spiritual spring clean and protection.

Remember, as you explore the unseen world, trust your intuition and always approach it with kindness and respect.

It's all in the mind

The bridge between our conscious minds and the realm of Dowsing lies in the extraordinary power of human consciousness. When Dowsing, we enter a unique "altered state"—a mindful mode where the chatter of the logical mind quiets, allowing us to tap into a deeper well of information.

This altered state is similar to the deep meditation achieved by seasoned Buddhist monks—a state that takes years of practice to cultivate. However, research suggests that experienced dowsers can access this profound level of focus within seconds.

The Science Behind the Art

Here's where things get fascinating: studies using EEG machines have shown that Dowsing synchronizes brainwave activity across both hemispheres. This is the holy grail for meditators—a state where Beta, Alpha, Theta, and Delta waves harmonize, creating a gateway to heightened awareness.

From a scientific perspective, Alpha, Theta, and Delta waves are associated with these "altered states." Children naturally experience these states more readily, which explains why they often take to Dowsing so easily. They haven't yet learned to overthink and analyze—they simply trust their intuition and "do it!"

This highlights the immense potential within each of us. Our minds hold incredible power, and when focused with intention, they can bridge the gap between the physical and extrasensory worlds. Science, through the principles of quantum physics, is starting to acknowledge the impact of human consciousness on the world around us.

Chapter 20

THE QUANTUM CONNECTION

The quantum world might sound like something out of *Alice in Wonderland*—no cause and effect, no linear time, and the ability of something to exist in two places at once. Yet, strangely enough, nothing in our reality can manifest without being "brought to life" by human consciousness. Scientists call this phenomenon "the Observer Effect."

In simpler terms, we are constantly interacting with unseen forces around us, and with focused intention, we have the power to shape our destinies. Thousands of experiments have validated the core tenets of quantum physics—the idea that our consciousness plays a mysterious role in creating the world we perceive.

The Interconnected Universe

Imagine our daily existence as a TV screen. The picture you see is made up of two realities: the image itself and the invisible frequencies carrying that image. By accessing these frequencies (through practices like Dowsing and Mindfulness), we can potentially change the "picture"—our reality.

Human consciousness serves as the bridge to this "Information Field," the Universal Mind, or whatever term resonates with you. Understanding the underlying science of the quantum world is crucial for both dowsers and those seeking to cultivate a strong Mindfulness practice.

Delving deeper into the quantum world might seem like a rabbit hole, but it's part of the intricate matrix we navigate as dowsers and mindful practitioners. The better we understand the

"Why" behind the practice, the more adept we become at harnessing its power.

The Power of the Right Brain

The universe is a vast consciousness, and everything within it resonates at its own unique frequency. From animals and plants to minerals, we are all interconnected through this universal field. Our individual frequencies form our energy bodies, which mirror our physical selves. Through practices like Dowsing, we can learn to connect with and understand this interconnectedness, even with the seemingly inanimate world around us.

The key player in this connection is our intuitive right brain. While our left brain handles logic and daily tasks, the right brain is the dreamer and the bridge to higher realities. Scientifically, the brain functions as two powerful computers: the left, a logical and detail-oriented realist, and the right, a creative and intuitive artist.

Here's a powerful quote that embodies this duality: "The intellect has little to do on the road to discovery; there comes a leap in consciousness—call it intuition or what you will—and the solution comes to you, and you don't know why or how." These words were spoken by none other than Albert Einstein, a testament to the power of our intuitive right brain.

Cultivating the Unconscious Mind

Our right brain is often the unsung hero. While the left brain gets the credit for managing our lives, the right brain is the silent conductor, handling millions of daily functions that keep us healthy. Moreover, it houses our unconscious mind, the vast reservoir that governs a staggering 90% of our daily existence.

To become strong psychics and mindful practitioners, we need to cultivate a relationship with our unconscious mind. It's a friend and ally, but it can also harbor past traumas and hidden memories that influence our present reality. These unseen forces can contribute to various health issues, but the good news is that through Dowsing and Mindfulness practices, we can explore and potentially heal these issues.

Now that you're well on your way to becoming a good dowser, let's step up a gear and see how you can become an *inspired* diviner. We do this by incorporating the art of Mindfulness. Once you get really familiar with its principles and practice, your Dowsing skills will enable you to achieve a unique and perfect meditation technique.

Everyday Dowsing For a Mindful You

Imagine a world where your intuition isn't just a fleeting feeling but a trusted guide woven into the fabric of your everyday life. That's the magic of everyday Dowsing, where the tools and techniques we've explored become companions on your journey to a more mindful and present existence. Let's ditch the grand pronouncements and hidden treasure hunts for a moment and focus on the practical applications of Dowsing that can elevate your daily routines and decisions.

The beauty of everyday Dowsing lies in its simplicity. You don't need to carve out dedicated hours for elaborate rituals. Instead, you can integrate Dowsing practices into your existing routines, transforming mundane tasks into mindful moments of self-discovery.

Mindful Grocery Mission

Standing bewildered in the cereal aisle, overwhelmed by the sugar-coated chaos? Instead of grabbing the first familiar box, pull out one L-rod and ask a simple question: "Take me to the cereal which is my healthiest option for today." As you give your (discreetly held) rod a little push, it will swing towards the row of cereal packets. Move forward slowly, and you will notice the rod gradually homing in on one particular brand. Finally, you will be in no doubt; this one in front of you is the selected target. You have been guided towards a more balanced choice while fostering a mindful approach to your dietary needs.

Dowsing Dress Dilemma

Facing a mountain of clothes, paralyzed by the "what to wear" conundrum? Don't waste precious time agonizing over outfits. Swing your pendulum into its search mode and point your index finger at your garments. As it moves along the rows, watch to see if your pendulum starts to gyrate. Do you get a 'Yes' for one particular outfit? When you do, your dilemma of what to wear is solved. This simple Dowsing practice can help you select clothing that supports your confidence and well-being throughout the day.

Dowsing Declutter Exercise

Feeling overwhelmed by untidy piles of stuff? Instead of aimlessly sorting through possessions, use your Dowsing tool to ask specific questions about each item. "Does this object spark joy?" or "Is it time to let this go?" The subtle movements of your Dowsing tool can guide your decluttering process, helping you clear your physical space and promote a sense of mental clarity.

Mindful Mealtime

We often eat on autopilot, barely savoring the flavors or appreciating the nourishment. Before digging into your meal, take a moment for mindful Dowsing. Hold your pendulum over your plate and ask: "Will this meal nourish me on all levels?" If the answer is no, you are being told to try something else. Change your menu and try again. This simple practice encourages a mindful approach to eating, helping you appreciate your food and fostering a healthy relationship with your body.

Decision-Making with Intuition

Stuck in a tough decision-making situation? Before making a rash choice, consider consulting your intuition. Formulate clear questions about your options, focusing on potential outcomes and long-term impacts. As before, get your pendulum to tell you Yes or No. The subtle movements of your Dowsing tool can offer a fresh perspective, helping you navigate tricky situations with greater clarity and confidence.

Everyday Dowsing isn't about achieving absolute certainty. It's about opening yourself to the whispers of your intuition and using them to make informed choices aligned with your well-being.

Chapter 21

JUST REMEMBER THIS...

Start Small: Don't overwhelm yourself with complex questions from the start. Begin with simple Yes-or-No questions related to everyday decisions. As you build trust in your intuition and the responses of your pendulum, L-rod, Y-rod, or bobber, you can gradually delve into more nuanced questions.

Remember the Mindfulness Connection: Both techniques—Dowsing and Mindfulness—can be complex, but I wanted to get you to a point where Dowsing is a natural part of your everyday life. Now we'll bring in Mindfulness and explore how you, as a dowser, can make Mindfulness your daily companion too.

Having incorporated Dowsing into your daily life, you'll find that your intuition becomes a trusted guide, helping you navigate everyday situations with greater ease and clarity. As you embrace these practices, you'll discover a deeper connection to yourself and the world around you, leading to a more mindful, present, and empowered existence.

You're Not Alone: As you venture deeper into the world of Dowsing, a sense of awe and wonder might wash over you. You're connecting with an ancient practice, tapping into the unseen forces that shape your reality, and unlocking the wisdom within your own intuition. But in these moments of exploration, it's important to remember one crucial truth: you're not alone.

The Dowsing community is a vibrant tapestry woven from individuals of all walks of life, united by a shared curiosity about the unseen and a desire to empower themselves through intuition.

This global tribe offers a sense of belonging, support, and shared experiences that enrich your Dowsing journey in countless ways.

Imagine attending a local Dowsing gathering, surrounded by fellow explorers eager to share their successes and challenges. You exchange stories, compare techniques, and learn from each other's experiences. Suddenly, that "Aha" moment you've been seeking clicks into place, sparked by a conversation with a colleague. This supportive network fosters a sense of camaraderie and shared purpose, propelling you forward.

But this is not the only way to connect with fellow enthusiasts. Online forums and communities offer a rich opportunity to engage with experienced dowsers worldwide. These platforms allow you to ask questions, share experiences, and gain valuable insights from those with years of practice. Whether you're new to Dowsing or have been practicing for a while, these virtual spaces are invaluable for continuous learning and personal growth. Just Google Dowsing organizations to get started.

And then there are Dowsing retreats, which provide a unique chance to immerse yourself in nature while connecting with fellow beginners and experienced mentors. Sharing your experiences offers advanced learning opportunities, the chance to share stories, and the potential to form lasting friendships. My Dowsing career took off when I attended a retreat with US divining legend Joey Korn. I joined eight other newcomers to the art at Joey's home in Augusta, Georgia, and spent a week learning about the unseen world of the subtle but powerful energies that are hidden behind all of life. Joey told us that with perseverance, we could unlock the secrets of the universe.

So when challenges arise—whether it's a pendulum spinning unexpectedly or L-rods refusing to move—reach out to your community. Fellow dowsers can offer advice, share similar experiences, and help you stay confident. Keep exploring new tools, trust in your intuition, and remember that the most exciting discoveries are still ahead.

PART 3
Chapter 22

YOUR JOURNEY INTO MINDFULNESS

What exactly is Mindfulness? Imagine Mindfulness as your personal key to unlocking the present moment. It's about being fully aware and engaged in what you are doing, feeling, and thinking right now. No more autopilot mode. No more letting life pass you by while your mind is caught up in the past or the future. Mindfulness brings you back to the here and now, allowing you to experience life more vividly and authentically.

Mindfulness isn't about achieving a blank mind or escaping reality. It's about embracing every moment with an open and accepting heart. Whether you're eating, walking, or simply breathing, Mindfulness turns these everyday activities into profound experiences. By practicing Mindfulness, you learn to observe your thoughts and feelings without judgment, creating a space where you can respond to life's challenges with clarity and compassion.

The Benefits of Practicing Mindfulness

You might be wondering, "Why should I practice Mindfulness?" Well, the benefits are truly transformative. Mindfulness has the power to enhance every aspect of your life. Let's dive into some of the incredible perks:

• **Reduced Stress and Anxiety:** Mindfulness helps you break free from the constant cycle of worry and stress. By grounding yourself in the present, you can alleviate anxiety and find a sense of calm.

• **Improved Focus and Concentration:** In a world filled with distractions, Mindfulness sharpens your ability to focus. Whether you're working, studying, or simply enjoying a hobby, Mindfulness helps you stay present and engaged.

• **Better Emotional Regulation:** Mindfulness teaches you to observe your emotions without being overwhelmed by them. This newfound awareness allows you to respond thoughtfully rather than react impulsively.

• **Enhanced Relationships:** By being fully present with others, Mindfulness fosters deeper connections and better communication. You'll find yourself more empathetic and understanding, improving your engagement with others.

• **Greater Resilience:** Life is full of ups and downs. Mindfulness builds your inner strength, helping you navigate challenges with grace and resilience.

Debunking Common Myths

As you begin your Mindfulness journey, it's important to clear up some common misconceptions that might be holding you back:

• **Myth:** Mindfulness is only for monks and yogis.

Reality: Mindfulness is for everyone. You don't need to live in a monastery or practice yoga to benefit from Mindfulness. It's a practical tool that anyone can use in everyday life.

• **Myth:** Mindfulness requires hours of meditation.

Reality: While meditation is a key component of Mindfulness, you don't need to meditate for hours. Even a few minutes of Mindfulness practice each day can make a significant difference.

• **Myth:** Mindfulness is about emptying your mind.

Reality: Mindfulness isn't about having a blank mind. It's about observing your thoughts and feelings without judgment. It's perfectly normal for your mind to wander; the key is to gently bring your focus back to the present.

• **Myth:** Mindfulness is a quick fix for all problems.

Reality: Mindfulness is not a magic cure. It's a practice that requires patience and consistency. Over time, it can lead to profound changes, but it's not an instant solution.

By understanding what Mindfulness truly is and dispelling these myths, you're setting a solid foundation for your journey. Remember, Mindfulness is a personal and transformative practice that grows with you. So, let's take the first steps together, and soon you'll discover the incredible power of living mindfully.

MINDFULNESS AND THE BRAIN

Mindfulness isn't just a fluffy concept; it has profound effects on the brain. Imagine your brain as a complex, interconnected network of highways. Mindfulness is like a master engineer, optimizing these highways for better traffic flow and communication.

When you practice Mindfulness, you engage specific areas of your brain, such as the prefrontal cortex and the anterior cingulate cortex. These regions are responsible for executive functions like decision-making, attention, and emotional regulation. Over time, regular Mindfulness practice can actually increase the density of grey matter in these areas, enhancing your cognitive abilities and emotional resilience.

But that's not all. Mindfulness also impacts the amygdala, the brain's alarm system that triggers the fight-or-flight response. Chronic stress can lead to an overactive amygdala, but Mindfulness helps to calm this response, reducing stress and anxiety levels.

Think of it as turning down the volume on your brain's alarm system, allowing you to respond to life's challenges with greater calm and clarity.

Moreover, Mindfulness strengthens the connections between different parts of the brain. This improved connectivity enhances overall brain function, promoting better integration of thoughts, emotions, and actions. It's like upgrading your brain's operating system, making it more efficient and harmonious.

Psychological and Physical Benefits

Psychological Benefits

1. **Reduced Anxiety and Depression:** Mindfulness helps you break free from the cycle of negative thinking, reducing symptoms of anxiety and depression. By focusing on the present moment, you can distance yourself from the worries and regrets that fuel these conditions.

2. **Emotional Regulation:** Mindfulness teaches you to observe your emotions without being swept away by them. This heightened awareness allows you to respond to emotional triggers more thoughtfully, reducing impulsivity and emotional reactivity.

3. **Improved Focus and Concentration:** In our multitasking world, it's easy to lose focus. Mindfulness sharpens your attention, helping you stay present and engaged in whatever you're doing. This enhanced concentration boosts productivity and effectiveness in all areas of life.

4. **Increased Self-Awareness:** Mindfulness encourages introspection and self-reflection. By becoming more aware of your thoughts, feelings, and behaviors, you gain valuable insights into your inner world, fostering personal growth and self-improvement.

Physical Benefits

• **Stress Reduction:** Chronic stress takes a toll on your body, leading to various health issues. Mindfulness reduces stress by calming the nervous system and lowering cortisol levels, promoting a sense of peace and relaxation.

• **Improved Sleep Quality:** Struggling with insomnia or restless nights? Mindfulness can help. By quieting the mind and promoting relaxation, Mindfulness practices enhance sleep quality, allowing you to wake up refreshed and rejuvenated.

• **Boosted Immune System:** Stress weakens the immune system, making you more susceptible to illness. Mindfulness bolsters immune function by reducing stress and promoting overall well-being, helping you stay healthy and resilient.

• **Pain Management:** Mindfulness has been shown to alleviate chronic pain by changing the way you perceive and respond to pain signals. By cultivating a non-judgmental awareness of pain, you can reduce its intensity and impact on your life.

Research and Studies Supporting Mindfulness

The benefits of Mindfulness are not just anecdotal; they are backed by a growing body of scientific research. Let's explore some key studies that highlight its effectiveness:

• **Mindfulness-Based Stress Reduction (MBSR):** Developed by Dr. Jon Kabat-Zinn, MBSR is one of the most well-known Mindfulness programs. Research shows that participants in MBSR programs experience significant reductions in stress, anxiety, and depression. They also report improvements in physical health and overall quality of life.

• **Mindfulness and Brain Structure:** A landmark study by Sara Lazar and her team at Harvard University found that just eight weeks of Mindfulness practice can lead to structural changes in the brain. Participants showed increased grey matter density in areas associated with learning, memory, and emotional regulation.

• **Mindfulness and Emotional Regulation:** Research published in *Frontiers in Human Neuroscience* demonstrates that Mindfulness practice enhances emotional regulation. Participants who practiced Mindfulness showed greater activation in brain regions involved in emotional control, helping them manage their emotions more effectively.

• **Mindfulness and Immune Function:** A study published in *Psychosomatic Medicine* found that Mindfulness meditation can enhance immune function. Participants who practiced Mindfulness showed increased activity in their immune system, suggesting a protective effect against illness and disease.

• **Mindfulness and Pain Management:** Research in the *Journal of Pain* highlights the effectiveness of Mindfulness in managing chronic pain. Participants who engaged in Mindfulness-based interventions reported reduced pain intensity and improved pain-related outcomes.

These studies, among many others, provide compelling evidence for the benefits of Mindfulness. By integrating Mindfulness into your daily life, you are not only enhancing your mental and physical well-being but also tapping into a scientifically validated practice with transformative potential.

Chapter 23

I MEDITATE, WHY DO I NEED MINDFULNESS?

If you meditate that's why you need Mindfulness! Do you really want to settle for second best? Mindfulness is meditation-plus. So, ignore that inner voice asking awkward questions, give it a go and then if it's not for you, no harm's been done.

Embarking on your Mindfulness journey begins with a simple yet profound step: setting your intentions. Think of intentions as your compass, guiding you towards a more mindful and fulfilling life. Without clear intentions, it's easy to lose direction and motivation. So, let's set the stage for success by defining your Mindfulness goals.

First, ask yourself, "Why do I want to practice Mindfulness?" Your reasons might be varied: reducing stress, improving focus, enhancing emotional well-being, or simply exploring a new way of being. Whatever your reasons, take a moment to write them down. This act of writing solidifies your intentions and serves as a reminder of your commitment when you're tempted (as we all are) to listen to that siren voice tempting us to slacken off.

Next, consider what you hope to achieve through Mindfulness. Are you looking to cultivate a sense of inner peace? Perhaps you want to develop better self-awareness or improve your relationships. Setting specific, achievable goals helps you stay focused and motivated. For instance, you might set an intention to practice mindful breathing for five minutes each day or to bring Mindfulness to your daily activities like eating or walking.

Remember, intentions are not rigid rules. They are gentle reminders of your aspirations, providing direction and purpose. Be kind to yourself and allow your intentions to evolve as you grow in your practice. Setting intentions is like planting seeds; with time and care, they will blossom into a beautiful Mindfulness practice.

Create a Mindful Environment

Now that you've set your intentions, it's time to create a space that nurtures your Mindfulness practice. Your environment plays a crucial role in supporting your journey, so let's transform your surroundings into a sanctuary of peace and presence.

Start by finding a quiet, comfortable location where you can practice Mindfulness without distractions. This could be a corner of your bedroom, a cozy spot in the living room, or even a peaceful outdoor setting. The key is to choose a place where you feel safe and relaxed.

Declutter your chosen space. A tidy environment helps to clear your mind and reduce distractions. Keep this area simple, with minimal furniture and decorations. Consider adding elements that promote a sense of calm, such as soft lighting, soothing colors, or natural elements like plants and flowers.

Incorporate Mindfulness tools that enhance your practice. A comfortable cushion or chair that supports your posture during meditation is essential. You might also use a timer to keep track of your practice sessions. Aromatherapy with essential oils like lavender or sandalwood can create a relaxing atmosphere, while gentle music or nature sounds can help you focus.

Make your Mindfulness space a place you look forward to visiting. Personalize it with items that inspire you, such as a favorite book, a journal for reflections, or a meaningful object like a crystal or a piece of artwork. By creating a mindful environment, you're setting the stage for a consistent and enjoyable practice.

Overcoming Initial Challenges

Starting a Mindfulness practice can be both exciting and daunting. It's natural to encounter challenges along the way, but with patience and perseverance, you can overcome them and build a strong foundation for your practice.

One common challenge is **restlessness**. Your mind might wander, and sitting still can feel uncomfortable. Remember, it's okay for you to lose concentration; this is part of the learning process. When you notice your mind drifting, gently bring your focus back to your breath or the present moment. Practice self-compassion. Yes, forgive yourself. The important thing is to keep going and not be tempted to give it all up in a bout of frustration.

Another challenge is **finding time for Mindfulness** in a busy schedule. Start small. Even a few minutes of Mindfulness each day can make a difference. Integrate Mindfulness into your daily routines, such as mindful eating, walking, or even brushing your teeth (more on this later). Gradually, you can increase the duration of your practice as it becomes a natural part of your life.

You might also face **resistance or doubt** about the effectiveness of Mindfulness. This is normal, especially when starting out. Keep an open mind and give yourself time to experience the benefits. Reading about others' experiences or joining a Mindfulness group can provide motivation and support.

Consistency is key. Establish a regular practice by setting a specific time each day for Mindfulness. Whether it's in the morning, during a lunch break, or before bed, find a time that works best for you and stick to it. Over time, this routine will become a cherished part of your day.

Finally, don't hesitate to seek guidance. Books, apps, online courses, and local classes can provide valuable resources and support. Consider finding a Mindfulness teacher or joining a community of like-minded individuals. Sharing your journey with others can offer encouragement and deepen your practice.

Remember, every step you take in your Mindfulness journey is progress. Embrace the challenges as opportunities to learn and grow. With dedication and an open heart, you'll discover the transformative power of Mindfulness, leading to a more peaceful and fulfilling life.

Well that's the What, now for the How

The breath is a powerful anchor that roots us in the present moment. Imagine it as a bridge, connecting the mind and body, linking the conscious with the subconscious. Breathing is something we do automatically, yet it holds immense potential when we bring our awareness to it.

Consider how your breath changes with your emotions: rapid and shallow when you're anxious, slow and deep when you're relaxed. By harnessing the power of your breath, you can influence your mental and emotional state. Mindful breathing is the key to unlocking this potential. It's about paying attention to each inhale and exhale, using the breath as a tool to cultivate Mindfulness.

Breathing mindfully grounds you in the here and now. It's a simple yet profound practice that calms the mind, soothes the nervous system, and brings clarity. In moments of stress or overwhelm, returning to your breath can be a sanctuary, a way to find peace amidst the chaos.

Chapter 24

BREATHE – IT'S SIMPLE, YOU'VE BEEN DOING IT ALL YOUR LIFE

Ready to experience the transformative power of breathing mindfully? Let's dive into some simple yet effective exercises that you can incorporate into your daily routine.

Mindful Breathing:

• Find a comfortable seated position. Close your eyes and take a few deep breaths, inhaling through your nose and exhaling through your mouth. Bring your attention to your natural breath. Notice the sensation of the air entering and leaving your nostrils. If your mind wanders, gently bring your focus back to your breath. Continue for 5-10 minutes.

The 4-7-8 Technique:

• Sit or lie down in a comfortable position. Close your eyes and inhale quietly through your nose for a count of four. Hold your breath for a count of seven. Exhale completely through your mouth for a count of eight. Repeat this cycle four times. This technique calms the nervous system and helps reduce stress.

Box Breathing:

• Sit up straight and exhale to empty your lungs. Inhale slowly through your nose to a count of four. Hold your breath for a count of four. Exhale through your mouth for a count of four. Hold your breath again for a count of four. Repeat for 4-5 minutes. Box breathing helps improve concentration and reduce anxiety.

Alternate Nostril Breathing (Nadi Shodhana):

• Sit comfortably and close your eyes. Use your right thumb to close your right nostril. Inhale deeply through your left nostril. Close your left nostril with your ring finger, release your thumb, and exhale through your right nostril. Inhale through your right nostril, close it with your thumb, and exhale through your left nostril. Continue alternating for 5-10 minutes. This exercise balances the mind and body.

These exercises are tools to help you connect with your breath and cultivate Mindfulness. Start with the one that resonates most with you and gradually explore the others.

Integrating Mindful Breathing into Daily Life

Mindful breathing isn't limited to formal practice; it can be seamlessly integrated into your daily life, enhancing your overall Mindfulness and well-being. Here's how to weave mindful breathing into everyday activities:

• **Morning Ritual:**

Begin your day with a few minutes of mindful breathing. Before you get out of bed, take a moment to focus on your breath. This sets a calm and centered tone for the day ahead.

• **During Transitions:**

Use transitions between activities as opportunities to practice mindful breathing. Whether you're moving from one meeting to another, commuting, or waiting in line (that's queueing for us Brits), take a few mindful breaths to reset and ground yourself.

• **Mindful Eating:**

Before you eat, take a moment to breathe mindfully. Notice the aroma, texture, and taste of your food. This practice not only enhances your Mindfulness but also improves your relationship with food.

- **Work Breaks:**

Incorporate short breathing exercises during your work breaks. A few minutes of mindful breathing can reduce stress, increase focus, and boost productivity.

- **Evening Wind-Down:**

Use mindful breathing to transition from the busyness of the day to a restful evening. Spend a few minutes focusing on your breath before bed to promote relaxation and improve sleep quality.

- **Mindful Movement:**

Integrate mindful breathing with physical activities like walking, yoga, or stretching. Coordinate your breath with your movements to enhance body awareness and create a meditative experience.

- **In Moments of Stress:**

When you feel stressed or overwhelmed, pause and take a few mindful breaths. This simple act can calm your nervous system and provide clarity, helping you respond to challenges more effectively.

By integrating mindful breathing into your daily routine, you create a consistent practice that supports your Mindfulness journey. These small moments of awareness accumulate, leading to profound changes in how you experience and navigate life. Remember, the breath is always with you, ready to anchor you in the present moment and bring a sense of peace and clarity.

Body Scan Meditation

Body awareness is the cornerstone of Mindfulness practice. It's about tuning into the sensations, signals, and rhythms of your body, fostering a deep connection with your physical self. Think of it as a dialogue between your mind and body, where you listen attentively to what your body has to say.

Often, we live in our heads, disconnected from our bodies. We rush through life, ignoring the subtle cues our bodies give us about stress, tension, or discomfort. By cultivating body awareness, you can break this cycle. You become attuned to the present moment, experiencing life through your senses and fostering a harmonious relationship with your body.

Body awareness helps you recognize patterns of tension and stress, allowing you to address them before they escalate. It also enhances your overall well-being by promoting relaxation, improving posture, and encouraging healthy habits. As you develop this awareness, you'll find that your body becomes a trusted ally in your Mindfulness journey, guiding you towards greater peace and balance.

Chapter 25

YES, BUT HOW DO I ACTUALLY DO IT?

Here's a step-by-step guide:

1 **Get Comfortable:**

Lie down on your back with your legs slightly apart and your arms resting by your sides, palms facing up. Alternatively, you can sit in a comfortable chair with your feet flat on the ground. Close your eyes and take a few deep breaths. Inhale through your nose, allowing your abdomen to rise, and exhale through your mouth, letting your body relax.

2 **Begin with Your Toes:**

Bring your attention to your toes. Notice any sensations—whether they are tingling, warm, or feel pressured. Simply observe without trying to change anything. Slowly shift your focus to the soles of your feet, then to your ankles. Continue this upward journey, moving your attention to your calves, knees, thighs, and so on. Spend a few moments on each area, observing any sensations that arise. As you scan each part of your body, you may notice areas of tension, discomfort, or even numbness. Acknowledge these sensations without judgment, allowing yourself to fully experience them.

3 **Breathe Into Areas of Tension:**

If you encounter areas of tension or discomfort, imagine directing your breath into those areas. Visualize the breath bringing relaxation and ease, softening any tightness. Gradually move your attention up through your torso, chest, shoulders, arms, and hands.

Finally, bring your focus to your neck, face, and head. Notice the sensations in each area, from the crown of your head to your forehead, eyes, cheeks, and jaws.

4 **Rest in Full-Body Awareness:**

Once you've scanned your entire body, take a moment to rest in this state of full-body awareness. Notice how your body feels as a whole, appreciating the sense of relaxation and connection.

5 **Gently Return:**

When you're ready, slowly bring your awareness back to your surroundings. Wiggle your fingers and toes, stretch gently, and open your eyes. Take a moment to reflect on your experience before resuming your normal activities.

Benefits of Body Scan

The body scan meditation offers numerous benefits, particularly in reducing stress and promoting relaxation. Let's explore how this practice can transform your well-being.

• **Stress Reduction:**

The body scan helps you identify and release tension stored in your body. By bringing awareness to areas of stress, you can consciously relax them, reducing overall stress levels. This practice activates the parasympathetic nervous system, which promotes a state of calm and relaxation.

• **Enhanced Relaxation:**

By systematically focusing on different parts of your body, the body scan induces a deep state of relaxation. It encourages the release of physical and mental tension, allowing you to unwind and recharge.

• **Improved Sleep:**

Regular practice of the body scan can improve sleep quality. By calming the mind and relaxing the body, this meditation helps you fall asleep more easily and enjoy more restful, restorative sleep.

- **Increased Self-Awareness:**

The body scan fosters a heightened sense of self-awareness. It helps you become more attuned to your body's needs, recognizing signals of fatigue, stress, or discomfort early on. This awareness empowers you to take proactive steps towards self-care and well-being.

- **Emotional Regulation:**

The practice of body scan meditation enhances emotional regulation. By observing sensations without judgment, you learn to acknowledge and accept your emotions as they are. This non-reactive approach cultivates emotional resilience and balance.

- **Mind-Body Connection:**

Finally, the body scan strengthens the connection between your mind and body. This integrated awareness promotes overall well-being, as you become more in tune with how your thoughts and emotions impact your physical state.

Incorporating body scan meditation into your routine is a powerful step towards reducing stress and enhancing relaxation. As you continue to practice, you'll discover a deeper connection with your body and a greater sense of peace and well-being. Remember, the journey of Mindfulness is unique for each individual, so be patient and compassionate with yourself as you explore this transformative practice.

MY BOSS IS A BULLY, CAN MINDFULNESS HELP ME?

Yes. Mindfulness can be an invaluable tool when preparing for and managing a difficult conversation, especially with someone like a bullying boss. Here's how you can use Mindfulness to approach the situation with clarity, calmness, and confidence:

Prepare with Mindfulness

• **Set an Intention:**

Before the conversation, take a moment to set a clear intention for what you want to achieve. Is your goal to express your concerns, set boundaries, or seek resolution? Setting an intention helps you stay focused during the conversation.

• **Center Yourself:**

Practice a few minutes of mindful breathing to center yourself. Close your eyes, take deep breaths, and focus on the rise and fall of your chest. This will help you calm any nerves and create a sense of inner stability.

• **Visualize the Outcome:**

Visualize the conversation going well. Imagine yourself speaking clearly and calmly, and envision your boss responding in a constructive manner. This positive visualization can help reduce anxiety and set a constructive tone for the conversation.

Stay Present During the Conversation

• **Practice Active Listening:**

When your boss is speaking, focus fully on their words without planning your response. This can prevent misunderstandings and help you respond more thoughtfully. If you find your mind wandering or becoming defensive, gently bring your focus back to their words and your breathing.

• **Manage Emotional Reactions:**

It's natural to feel a surge of emotion, especially when dealing with someone you find intimidating. If you notice anger, frustration, or fear arising, acknowledge the feeling without letting it control your behavior. Take a deep breath, feel your feet on the ground, and remind yourself of your intention for the conversation.

- **Pause Before Responding:**

Mindfulness teaches us the power of the pause. Before responding to something your boss says, take a brief moment to collect your thoughts. This pause can prevent reactive or defensive replies and allows you to respond with clarity and composure.

Communicate Mindfully

- **Speak Clearly and Calmly:**

When it's your turn to speak, do so slowly and deliberately. Keep your tone even and your words clear. If you feel overwhelmed, take a deep breath before continuing. Mindful speech helps to convey your message effectively and reduces the chance of escalating tensions.

- **Set Boundaries Respectfully:**

If your boss's behavior crosses a line, use Mindfulness to assert your boundaries calmly. For example, you might say, "I feel uncomfortable when you speak to me in that way. I'd appreciate it if we could discuss this respectfully." The key is to remain firm but not aggressive.

- **Stay Focused on Facts:**

Stick to the facts rather than getting drawn into emotional arguments. Mindfulness can help you stay grounded and focused on the specific issues at hand rather than getting caught up in personal attacks or defensiveness.

Mindfulness Techniques to Use

- **Grounding Exercise:**

During the conversation, if you start to feel overwhelmed, discreetly press your feet into the floor and feel the contact with the ground. This grounding technique can help you stay present and prevent your mind from spiraling.

- **Breathing Techniques:**

Focus on deep, slow breaths, especially if your boss says something triggering. A simple technique is to inhale for a count of four, hold for a count of four, and exhale for a count of four. This will help calm your nervous system.

- **Mantra or Affirmation:**

Having a mantra or affirmation can help maintain your focus and confidence. For example, silently repeating, "I am calm and in control," can reinforce your inner strength.

Reflect After the Conversation

- **Practice Self-Compassion:**

After the conversation, take time to reflect on how it went. Regardless of the outcome, practice self-compassion. Acknowledge that difficult conversations are challenging and that you did your best under the circumstances.

- **Learn and Adjust:**

Reflect on what worked well and what didn't. Use these insights to adjust your approach for future interactions. Mindfulness helps you approach this reflection without judgment, allowing you to learn and grow from the experience.

Managing a difficult conversation with a boss you regard as a bully is never easy, but Mindfulness equips you with tools to handle it with grace and confidence. By preparing mindfully, staying present, communicating clearly, and reflecting with self-compassion, you can navigate the conversation in a way that protects your well-being and upholds your self-respect. Remember, Mindfulness is about staying connected to the present moment, which helps you remain composed and effective, even in challenging situations.

Chapter 26

ARE YOU MAKING A MEAL OF MINDFULNESS? GOOD!

Eating is a daily ritual, yet it's often performed on autopilot. Imagine transforming your meals into moments of **Mindfulness**, where each bite becomes a celebration of the present moment. As you look at your food, appreciate its colors, textures, and aromas. Notice the intricate details that you might usually overlook.

Think about what you are putting on your fork, savor the flavor as you chew, be aware of your surroundings, and look at what else is on your plate. Contemplate where the vegetables might have been grown, their journey from farm to fork. Perhaps take a moment of silent gratitude for your good fortune to have enough to eat, when so many others are less fortunate. Chew thoroughly and pay attention to how the food feels in your mouth. Notice the subtle changes in taste and texture as you continue to chew.

As you eat, put down your utensils between bites. This simple act slows down the pace of eating and allows you to fully engage with the experience. Practicing **Mindfulness** while eating not only enhances your appreciation of food but also fosters a healthier relationship with what you consume. By the way, avoid distractions such as TV, smartphones, or multitasking. Focus solely on the act of eating. By doing so, you transform a routine activity into a meditative practice, fostering a deeper connection with your body and the present moment.

Mindful Walking and Movement

Walking is another everyday activity that can be enriched with Mindfulness. **Mindful walking** involves bringing your full attention to the experience of walking, turning it into a moving meditation. It's a beautiful way to integrate **Mindfulness** into your daily life while reaping the benefits of physical activity.

Start by choosing a quiet place where you can walk undisturbed. Begin with a few deep breaths to ground yourself in the present moment. As you start to walk, notice the sensation of your feet touching the ground. Pay attention to the movement of your legs, the shifting of your weight, and the rhythm of your steps.

Feel the muscles in your legs and the way your arms swing naturally. Notice the gentle rise and fall of your breath as you walk. Let your senses come alive, taking in the sights, sounds, and smells around you.

If your mind starts to wander, gently bring your attention back to the act of walking. You can use a simple phrase like "left, right" to anchor your mind to your steps. **Mindful walking** is not about reaching a destination; it's about fully experiencing the journey.

You can also practice **Mindfulness** during other forms of movement, such as stretching, yoga, or even daily chores. The key is to bring your full attention to the physical sensations and movements of your body. This practice not only enhances physical awareness but also cultivates a deep sense of presence and tranquility.

Routine Tasks

Yes, they often feel mundane, but routine tasks offer perfect opportunities to practice **Mindfulness**. By bringing mindful awareness to these activities, you transform them into moments of calm and clarity.

Take washing the dishes, for example. Instead of rushing through it, approach it with **Mindfulness**. Feel the warm water on your hands, notice the texture of the soap, and listen to the sound of running water. Focus on each dish individually, paying attention to the process of cleaning it. This turns a simple chore into a peaceful, meditative experience.

Another example is brushing your teeth. Feel the sensation of the toothbrush against your teeth and gums, notice the taste of the toothpaste, and the rhythmic motion of your hand. Be fully present in the moment, appreciating the care you're giving to your oral health.

Mindfulness can also be applied to tasks like folding laundry, sweeping the floor, or making the bed. Engage your senses fully, paying attention to the textures, movements, and sounds involved in each task. This is how you cultivate **Mindfulness** that permeates your daily life.

The goal with these routine tasks is to slow down and focus on the present moment, letting go of any desire to rush or multitask. Embrace each activity with a sense of curiosity and appreciation. Over time, you'll find that these mindful moments accumulate, creating a more peaceful and centered way of living.

Incorporating **Mindfulness** into everyday activities doesn't require extra time; it simply involves a shift in awareness. By practicing **Mindfulness** while eating, walking, and performing routine tasks, you weave **Mindfulness** into the fabric of your daily life.

Chapter 27

NOW LET'S GET EMOTIONAL

Emotions are an integral part of the human experience, yet we often struggle to understand and manage them. Imagine emotions as waves in the ocean: they rise, peak, and eventually subside. By recognizing and understanding these emotional waves, we can navigate them with greater ease and grace.

Start by paying attention to your emotional state throughout the day. Notice the subtle shifts in your mood and how different situations trigger various emotions. Are you feeling joy, sadness, anger, or fear? Acknowledge these feelings without judgment, as if you were an impartial observer.

To deepen your understanding, explore the physical sensations associated with your emotions. For instance, where do you feel tension when you're anxious? How does your body react when you're happy? This practice helps you connect with your emotions on a somatic level, fostering a more holistic awareness.

Naming your emotions can also be incredibly powerful. When you label what you're feeling, you bring clarity to your emotional landscape. It's like shining a light in a dark room, allowing you to see things more clearly. For example, instead of saying, "I feel bad," try specifying, "I feel frustrated" or "I feel overwhelmed." This specificity enhances your emotional literacy and empowers you to address your feelings more effectively.

Understanding your emotions involves recognizing their transient nature. Emotions come and go, and no single feeling defines you. By observing your emotions mindfully, you create a space where you can respond thoughtfully rather than react impulsively, fostering emotional balance and resilience—which brings confidence.

Techniques for Managing Stress and Anxiety

Stress and anxiety are common companions in modern life, but **Mindfulness** offers effective techniques for managing these challenges. Here's a few more practical ways to cultivate a sense of calm and control even in the face of stress.

• **Grounding Exercises:** Grounding techniques help anchor you in the present moment, reducing anxiety. One effective method is the 5-4-3-2-1 exercise: identify five things you can see, four things you can touch, three things you can hear, two things you can smell, and one thing you can taste. This sensory focus draws your attention away from anxious thoughts and grounds you in the here and now.

• **Mindful Movement:** Engage in mindful movement practices such as yoga, tai chi, or simply stretching. Focus on the sensations in your body as you move, paying attention to your breath and the rhythm of your movements. This practice not only reduces stress but also enhances physical and mental well-being.

• **Visualization:** Use visualization to create a mental sanctuary. Close your eyes and imagine a peaceful place where you feel safe and relaxed. It could be a beach, a forest, or any other calming setting. Spend a few minutes immersing yourself in this visualization, noticing the sights, sounds, and sensations. Visualization helps reduce stress by evoking a sense of tranquility.

By incorporating these techniques into your daily routine, you can effectively manage stress and anxiety, fostering a more balanced state of mind.

Cultivate Some Compassion—For Yourself

Mindfulness isn't just about awareness; it's also about developing a compassionate and accepting attitude toward yourself as well as others. Embracing compassion and self-acceptance can transform your relationship with you.

Start by deciding that you are not going to be so hard on yourself. When you make a mistake or face a challenging situation, treat yourself with the same kindness and understanding you would offer a friend. Acknowledge your imperfections and remind yourself that it's okay not to be perfect. Accept that everyone makes mistakes and that these experiences are part of being human.

To nurture compassion, try some **loving-kindness meditation**. Begin by sitting comfortably and closing your eyes. Take a few deep breaths to center yourself. Then, silently repeat phrases like, "May I be happy, may I be healthy, may I be safe, may I live with ease." As you repeat these phrases, imagine sending these wishes to yourself.

Then, extend these wishes to others. Start with someone you care about, then move to a neutral person, and finally to someone with whom you have difficulty. This practice helps to expand your circle of compassion and fosters a sense of interconnectedness.

Practice self-acceptance by embracing your thoughts and feelings without judgment. Recognize that it's okay to experience a range of emotions and that you don't need to suppress or deny them. Acceptance involves acknowledging your current experience without striving to change it. This attitude of acceptance creates a safe space for you to explore your inner world and promotes emotional healing.

Reflect on your strengths and accomplishments regularly. Celebrate your achievements, *no matter how small they may seem.*

This practice reinforces a positive self-image and encourages a more compassionate relationship with yourself.

By cultivating compassion and self-acceptance, you create a supportive inner environment where you can thrive. This foundation of kindness and understanding not only enhances your Mindfulness practice but will also enrich your quality of life.

As you continue to develop emotional awareness through recognizing and understanding emotions, managing stress and anxiety, and cultivating compassion and self-acceptance, you'll find yourself more equipped to navigate the complexities of life with grace and resilience.

Chapter 28

KNOWLEDGE SPEAKS, WISDOM LISTENS

Relationships are the heart of the human experience, and Mindfulness can profoundly enhance how we connect and communicate with others. Try being fully present in every conversation, deeply listening, and responding with clarity and empathy. This level of engagement transforms interactions and fosters genuine connections.

So, when someone is speaking to you, give them your undivided attention. Put away distractions, maintain eye contact, and truly listen to their words, tone, and body language. Resist the urge to interrupt or plan your response while they're talking. Instead, focus on understanding their perspective and feelings.

Reflect back what you've heard to show that you're listening. Simple phrases like "What I'm hearing is..." or "It sounds like you're feeling..." can confirm that you've understood their message. This not only validates their experience but also builds trust and rapport.

Practice non-judgmental awareness in conversations. Avoid jumping to conclusions or making assumptions about what the other person is saying. Approach each interaction with an open mind and a genuine curiosity about their viewpoint. This openness creates a safe space for honest and meaningful dialogue.

Mindfulness in Interactions

Mindfulness in interactions means being fully present and attentive in every encounter. It's about bringing the same level of awareness and presence to your social interactions as you do to your meditation practice. Here are more tips for how you can cultivate this skill:

• **Pause and Center Yourself:** Before entering a conversation, take a moment to pause and center yourself. Take a few deep breaths to ground yourself in the present moment. This prepares you to engage mindfully and with intention.

• **Listen with Your Whole Being:** Don't just listen with your ears. Use your whole being. Pay attention to your companion's words, tone, and body language. Notice the emotions and intentions behind their words. This deep listening fosters empathy and understanding.

• **Respond Thoughtfully:** When it's your turn to speak, respond thoughtfully. Take a moment to reflect on what you've heard before replying. Your responses should be considerate and project your genuine understanding of their perspective.

• **Practice Patience:** Patience is key in mindful interactions. Allow the other person to express themselves fully without rushing them or finishing their sentences. Patience creates a space for deeper and more meaningful exchanges. You'll be surprised how, just by listening, you'll gain a reputation for being a wonderful conversationalist!

• **Manage Your Emotions:** Be aware of your own feelings during interactions. If you feel triggered or upset, take a moment to breathe and regain your composure before responding. Mindful awareness of your emotions helps you stay in command of the conversation.

If you follow this guidance you'll transform everyday conversations into opportunities for deeper connection and understanding which will enrich your social life and foster a greater sense of community.

Building Stronger, More Compassionate Relationships

Mindfulness nurtures compassion. When you approach your relationships with compassion, you create a nurturing environment where both you and your loved ones can thrive.

I've already mentioned this, but it bears repeating: Start by cultivating self-compassion. Treat yourself with the same kindness and understanding you would offer a close friend. When you make mistakes, acknowledge your frailty without harsh judgment. This self-compassion forms the basis for extending compassion to others.

And, practice empathy which involves putting yourself in the other person's shoes and understanding their feelings and experiences. When your partner or friend shares something with you, try to feel what they're feeling and see the world from their perspective. This empathy fosters deep emotional bonds and mutual respect.

Engage in **loving-kindness meditation** to enhance your capacity for compassion. Sit comfortably, close your eyes, and bring to mind someone you care about. Silently repeat phrases like, "May you be happy, may you be healthy, may you be safe, may you live with ease." Doing this softens your heart and promotes a caring attitude.

Mindful presence is another key to building compassionate relationships. Show up fully for your loved ones, offering your undivided attention and genuine presence. When spending time together, focus on the moment rather than letting your mind wander to other concerns. This presence communicates love and care and strengthens your bond.

And communicate with kindness and honesty. Mindfulness helps you express yourself authentically while remaining considerate of the other person's feelings. Avoid harsh words or criticism, and instead, use "I" statements to share your experiences and needs. For example, say, "I feel upset when..." rather than "You always...".

Lastly, and certainly not least, practice **forgiveness**. Holding onto grudges and resentments harms your relationships and yourself. Mindfulness helps you let go of past hurts and approach conflicts with a fresh perspective. Forgiveness doesn't mean condoning harmful behavior but rather freeing yourself from the burden of negative emotions.

By integrating Mindfulness into your relationships, you build a foundation of compassion, empathy, and genuine connection. These qualities create a supportive, loving environment where relationships can flourish. As you continue to develop Mindfulness in your communication, interactions, and relationships, you'll discover a deeper sense of connection and fulfillment and, as a bonus, emotional well-being.

Chapter 29

MINDFULNESS, I LOVE IT...BUT I MUST DO THIS FIRST

Distractions, restlessness, and something called "displacement activity" are common hurdles to pursuing Mindfulness. There are times when the spirit is willing but the flesh is weak. We just don't feel like disciplining ourselves to clear the decks, put aside all distractions, and settle down to an hour of doing nothing. However, recognizing and addressing these obstacles is part of your journey, and the more you make your meditations a habit, the less you'll have to fight the siren voices in your head.

Start by acknowledging that distractions are normal. The goal is not to eliminate distractions but to develop a gentle awareness of them. When you notice your mind wandering, calmly bring your focus back to your breath or the present activity. This act of returning to the present moment is itself a valuable part of the practice.

Retreat to your dedicated space, your comfortable spot where you can sit or lie down without interruption, and tell family members or housemates about your practice to minimize disturbances.

If restlessness is a persistent problem, start with a shorter session and gradually increase the duration as you become more comfortable with your routine. Incorporate mindful movement like yoga or walking meditation to channel restlessness into purposeful activity. Movement can help settle the mind and prepare you for stillness.

If you find yourself frequently distracted, try using a focus point, such as a candle flame or a soothing object, to anchor your attention. Guided meditations can also provide structure and help maintain focus, especially for beginners.

Remember, patience and kindness toward yourself are essential. Each time you bring your attention back from a distraction, you strengthen your Mindfulness muscle. Over time, this becomes easier and more natural.

Expectations and Frustrations

Embarking on a Mindfulness journey often comes with certain expectations. You might hope for immediate peace, profound insights, or dramatic changes in your life. That is a rare manifestation! Most beginners struggle, sometimes to the point of giving up (just like dowsers haunted by the Cosmic Joker). But there will be less threat of that for you if you manage your expectations. Mindfulness ALWAYS works, but you may not be aware of its working at the time.

Just as physical exercise strengthens muscles over time, Mindfulness practice builds your mental muscles in the same way. Avoid setting rigid goals or expecting quick fixes. Instead, appreciate each moment of practice as it comes.

Frustration can arise when your experience doesn't match your expectations. You might feel discouraged if your mind remains busy or if you don't feel immediate benefits. When frustration arises, just observe the feeling, understand its origins, and let it pass.

Shift your focus from outcomes to the process. Celebrate small victories, like noticing a moment of calm or catching yourself in mid-mindful breath. These small moments accumulate and build confidence.

As ever, treat yourself with the same kindness you would offer a friend facing similar challenges. Remember that everyone's Mindfulness journey is unique, and comparing yourself with others can hinder your progress. Embrace your personal path.

Lastly, maintain a beginner's mind. Approach each practice session as if it's your first, free from preconceived notions and judgments. This mindset fosters openness and receptivity, allowing you to fully engage with the present.

Keep On Keeping On

Especially in the early weeks, sustaining motivation in your **Mindfulness** practice can be particularly challenging. Here's a reminder of strategies that will help you stay committed and inspired on your journey:

• **Set Realistic Goals:** Begin with manageable ambitions that fit your lifestyle. Whether it's a few minutes of mindful breathing each morning or a weekly meditation session, setting achievable targets helps build consistency and confidence.

• **Create a Routine:** Establish a regular practice time that fits naturally into your daily schedule. Consistency reinforces habit formation and makes Mindfulness an integral part of your life. Whether it's the first thing in the morning or before bedtime, find a time that works best for you.

• **Join a Community:** Engage with a Mindfulness group or find a meditation buddy. Practicing with others provides support, accountability, and shared experiences. Online forums, local classes, or virtual meetups can connect you with like-minded individuals.

• **Reflect on Your Progress:** Keep a journal to track your experiences and reflections. Note the challenges you face, the insights you gain, and the changes you observe in your thoughts and behaviors. Reflecting on your journey can provide motivation and reassure you that you are growing.

• **Incorporate Variety:** Explore different Mindfulness practices to keep your routine fresh and engaging. Try various forms of meditation, mindful movement, or breathing exercises. This variety prevents monotony and helps you discover what resonates most with you.

• **Stay Inspired:** Read books, listen to podcasts, or watch videos about Mindfulness and meditation. Learning from experienced practitioners and teachers can provide fresh perspectives and inspiration. Surround yourself with resources that uplift and motivate you.

Remember, the journey is as important as the destination. Embrace each step with curiosity, patience, and kindness, knowing that every moment of Mindfulness contributes to your overall well-being and growth.

Chapter 30

WE ALL NEED SOME OF THIS

Some of what? **Loving-kindness**, of course. And, ever ready to oblige with something relevant to our needs, Mindfulness has a meditation, also known as **Metta**, to help us cultivate compassion and unconditional love toward ourselves and others. Imagine sending waves of warmth and kindness from your heart, enveloping yourself, your loved ones, and even those you find challenging. This practice not only enhances your emotional well-being but also fosters a deep sense of interconnectedness.

Begin by sitting comfortably and closing your eyes. Take a few deep breaths to center yourself. Start by directing loving-kindness toward yourself. Silently repeat phrases like, "May I be content. May I be healthy. May I be safe. May I live with serenity." Allow these words to resonate within you, filling your heart with warmth and compassion.

Next, extend these wishes to someone you care about. Visualize this person and silently repeat the phrases, sending them your heartfelt wishes. Gradually, extend your loving-kindness to neutral individuals, those you have difficulty with, and finally to all beings everywhere. This practice can transform your heart, nurturing compassion and empathy for all humans everywhere.

Visualization Techniques

Visualization is a powerful tool in Mindfulness, allowing you to create a mental sanctuary that promotes peace and relaxation. Think of it as painting a vivid picture in your mind, a place where you can retreat to find solace and rejuvenation.

Start by finding a quiet place to sit or lie down. Close your eyes and take a few deep breaths. Begin to imagine a peaceful scene, like a tranquil beach, a serene forest, or a cozy room. Engage all your senses to make this visualization as vivid as possible. Feel the warmth of the sun, hear the gentle rustle of leaves, and smell the fresh air.

Spend a few minutes immersing yourself in this mental imagery. Whenever you feel stressed or overwhelmed, return to this mental sanctuary to find calm and clarity. Visualization techniques can also be used for setting intentions, achieving goals, and healing. By regularly practicing visualization, you enhance your ability to focus, relax, and manifest positive outcomes.

Gratitude Practices

Gratitude is a profound aspect of Mindfulness that shifts your focus from what's lacking in your life to the abundance you have around you compared with many others. Feeling gratitude nurtures a positive mindset, enhances well-being, and fosters a deeper appreciation for the present moment.

Start by keeping a gratitude journal. Each day, write down three to five things you are grateful for. These can be simple pleasures, acts of kindness, or significant achievements. Reflect on these entries regularly, allowing the feelings of gratitude to fill you.

Try the **Gratitude Pause**. Throughout your day, take moments to pause and silently acknowledge something you are thankful for. It could be the warmth of the sun, the support of a friend, or a delicious meal. These small moments of gratitude accumulate, creating a habit.

Integrate gratitude into your Mindfulness by ending your meditation sessions with a few minutes of reflecting on what you

are grateful for. This reinforces positive emotions and deepens your
Mindfulness journey.

GROW UP!

Yes, that's what you are now doing. You're growing upwards,
becoming a new, better person. For this chapter, start by reflecting
on what truly matters to you. What are your core values? How
do you want to grow? Write down your goals, ensuring they are
specific, measurable, attainable, relevant, and time-bound (be
SMART).

Mindful goal setting involves aligning your aspirations with
your values and focusing on the process rather than just the
outcome. It's about setting intentions that nurture your growth and
well-being.

Next, break these goals into smaller, manageable steps. This
makes them less overwhelming and more achievable. Regularly
review and adjust your goals, celebrating progress and learning
from setbacks. Approach your goals with a sense of curiosity and
openness, allowing flexibility in how you achieve them.

Journaling

This habit is a powerful tool for self-discovery and personal
growth. It provides a safe space to explore your thoughts, emotions,
and experiences, fostering greater self-awareness and clarity.

Begin by setting aside a few minutes each day to write. You can
start with prompts like, "Today I feel...," "I am grateful for...," or "A
challenge I faced today was...." Allow your writing to flow freely
without judgment or censorship. This practice helps you process
emotions, identify patterns, and gain insights into your inner
world.

Practices, such as end-of-day reflections or weekly reviews,
deepen your self-awareness. At the end of each day, take a few

minutes to reflect on your experiences. What went well? What did you learn? How can you improve? These reflections guide your personal growth and enhance your Mindfulness practice. Can you see now that you're no longer on autopilot? That's Mindfulness!

Embracing Change

Mindfulness teaches us that change is a natural part of life. Embracing change and growth with a mindful attitude involves accepting impermanence and viewing challenges as opportunities for development.

Cultivate a **growth mindset** by seeing failures and setbacks as learning experiences. When faced with change, practice acceptance and openness. Acknowledge your emotions and thoughts without judgment, allowing yourself to adapt and grow. Embrace change by staying present and engaged in the process. Rather than resisting or fearing change, approach it with curiosity and a sense of adventure. This mindset transforms challenges into stepping stones.

Chapter 31

DO YOU FEEL YOU'RE BECOMING A MINDFUL YOU?

A reminder: becoming a **Mindful you** involves integrating Mindfulness into your daily life. Establishing a routine helps make it a natural and consistent part of your day.

Start by setting aside specific times for Mindfulness practice. Whether it's in the morning, during lunch breaks, or before bed, find a time that works best for you. Begin with short sessions and gradually increase the duration as you become more comfortable.

Incorporate Mindfulness into everyday activities. Practice mindful eating, walking or even (yes, I know I've said it before) brushing your teeth! These small moments accumulate, enhancing your overall awareness and well-being.

Be patient and flexible with your routine. Life can be unpredictable, and it's okay to adjust your routine as needed. The key is consistency and commitment.

Resources and Support

There are numerous tools and communities available to guide and support you. As I said earlier, explore books, apps, and online courses. These resources offer valuable insights, techniques, and guided practices. Apps like **Headspace**, **Calm**, and **Insight Timer** provide a variety of guided meditations and exercises.

Consider joining a group or finding a meditation buddy. Local classes, online forums, and virtual meetups connect you with like-minded individuals. And don't be too shy to seek guidance from experienced teachers or mentors who can offer personalized advice, answer your questions, and provide support as you navigate your path.

Continuing Your Quest

Mindfulness is a lifelong adventure with profound long-term benefits. As you continue your practice, you'll notice improvements in your mental, emotional, and physical well-being. Long-term practice enhances emotional regulation, reduces stress, and increases resilience. It fosters greater self-awareness, compassion, and empathy, enriching your relationships and overall quality of life. What's not to like?

Some Final Reflections

Well, that's almost it for this basic guide to Mindfulness (but don't go away as the best is yet to come). Take a moment to reflect on your journey so far. We've covered a heck of a lot of ground. Consider the progress you've made, the challenges you've overcome, and the insights you've gained.

Reflect on how Mindfulness has impacted your life. What positive changes have you noticed? How has your awareness, emotional well-being, and overall quality of life improved? Celebrate these milestones and acknowledge the effort you've put into your practice.

Recognize that Mindfulness is an ongoing journey. There will always be new experiences, challenges, and opportunities for growth. Embrace each moment with curiosity and openness, knowing that your practice will continue to evolve.

And as you continue your exploration, know that you are not alone. There is a vast community of individuals on the same path, and countless resources to support you. Embrace a Mindful life. Let it guide you toward greater peace, joy, and fulfillment. Your journey is unique, and every step you take brings you closer to a more meaningful existence. And thank you for embarking on this journey with me. And a special Thank you if you now stay with me to learn how to make your Mindfulness practice unique to you.

PART 4
Chapter 32

HAVE A CLOSE BRUSH WITH MINDFULNESS TWICE A DAY

First, allow me to reassure you, Mindfulness doesn't require a dramatic upheaval to your life. Forget any visions of mountain retreats and silent meditation sessions (although these are perfectly valid)—as you will know by now you can cultivate a mindful routine right in the heart of your everyday activities.

For instance, is brushing your teeth now a sensory experience? Are you feeling the cool water on your skin, the texture of the bristles, the minty freshness in your mouth? Are you noticing the sound of the running water and the subtle movements involved in brushing your teeth and gums?

This same approach applies to seemingly mundane activities like walking. Instead of getting lost in thought, are you aware of your body's movements? Do you feel the ground beneath your feet, the rhythm of your steps, and the way your breath moves in and out? Are you registering the sights, sounds, and smells around you—a chirping bird, a blooming flower, the warmth of the sun?

And what about eating? In our fast-paced world, meals often become rushed affairs, eaten on the go or while multitasking. But you're not like that, are you? You've learned to slow down and savor the experience. You're noticing the colors and textures of your food, the aroma that fills your senses. You're taking your time, chewing slowly, appreciating the flavor and texture of every mouthful.

While washing the dishes, you're focusing on the feel of warm water on your skin, the sound of the clinking dishes, and the simple act of cleaning. And with the laundry, you're now noticing the weight of the fabric and the smooth folds you create.

Remember, Mindfulness isn't about achieving some perfect state of zen; it's about cultivating a present-moment awareness that enriches your everyday experience. You know to start small, be patient, and watch the magic unfold in your life.

Now, let's bring our Dowsing skills to bear and turbo-charge our Mindfulness experience.

Finding Our Inner Oasis (With Trusted Dowsing Tool in Hand)

Now that we've explored the fascinating worlds of Dowsing and Mindfulness, and awakened the Dowsing superpower within us, it's time to understand how combining these practices can provide a unique gateway to a more mindful and serene life.

But before I get to that, a quick practicality: Don't forget that the simplest form of Dowsing is the binary **Yes/No** question. If you're asking When? Why? Who? What? Where? Which? You need to give your pendulum a series of options to drill down to the final **Yes/No** answer. For example, **What's caused my current mood of anxiety? A health issue? A relationship problem? That conversation I had at the bus stop?** You'll always have to make suggestions unless, of course, you are adept with the Dowsing chart.

Back to the magic of Dowsing as a Mindfulness gateway. Imagine this: you are standing amidst a bustling farmers' market, overwhelmed by the vibrant stalls overflowing with fresh produce. You discreetly hold one L-rod, focusing your mind on a single question: "Which fruits and vegetables will nourish me most today?" As the L-rod points you toward a particular stall, a sense of calm washes over you. You're no longer lost in the sensory overload but present in the moment, actively participating in your own well-being.

Dowsing isn't just about finding hidden objects or answering yes-or-no questions. It's about cultivating a state of mindful awareness, sharpening your focus, and tuning into the subtle energy around you. The act of Dowsing itself demands a quiet mind and a clear intention. You must be present in the moment to formulate your question, hold the tool with focus, and interpret its subtle movements. In this way, Dowsing becomes a powerful Mindfulness exercise in its own right, training your brain to quieten the mental chatter and connect with the present experience.

Chapter 33

DON'T STOP NOW, THE BEST IS YET TO COME

You might be wondering, "Why do I need this next section? I've learned about Dowsing, and I'm a Mindfulness practitioner—so why should I read on?" The answer is simple: because you don't want to settle for good when you can achieve excellence.

Think of it like this—when I first learned Pitman's shorthand years ago, my tutor told me that to truly master it, I needed to learn the basics first and then I would know enough to discover a different, more advanced way of doing it! The same principle applies here. By integrating Dowsing with Mindfulness, you're not just practicing two separate disciplines—you're creating a unique and powerful meditation routine that's perfectly suited to you in the context of the frenetic world we live in.

Let's go.

Imagine unlocking a deeper level of awareness and insight, a synergy that enhances and amplifies the benefits of both practices. Dowsing connects us to subtle energies and insights beyond our conscious mind, while Mindfulness grounds us in the present moment, fostering a deep sense of awareness and calm. Together, these practices create a powerful tool for self-discovery and personal growth.

Think of Dowsing and Mindfulness as two sides of the same coin. Dowsing brings clarity to your intuitive senses, while Mindfulness ensures you remain grounded and present to fully experience these insights. Not only will you become more aware of your thoughts and emotions, but you'll also gain a deeper understanding of the underlying energies influencing them. This comprehensive awareness fosters a stronger connection with the world around you.

Setting Intentions and Practical Integration

Before embarking on this combined modality, it's crucial to set clear intentions. Start by reflecting on what you want to achieve—greater clarity, emotional balance, spiritual growth? Whatever your goals, jot them down. This solidifies your intentions and serves as a constant reminder of your commitment.

Next, consider how you'll integrate these practices into your daily life. Set realistic, achievable objectives. For example, you might use a pendulum to select the best time for your meditation or to check your energy levels before and after the session. This keeps you focused and motivated.

Remember, intentions are flexible guides, not rigid rules. Be open to adjusting them as you progress. Approach your practice with curiosity, allowing your intentions to evolve with your experiences. By having clear and heartfelt ambitions, you create a strong foundation for what's ahead.

Now that you've laid the groundwork, let's explore the practicalities.

Getting Into the Swing Of Things

Before starting your session, establish a mindful mindset. Ask your pendulum, "What is my appropriate state of mind to achieve the optimum benefit from my meditation? Calmness? Alert focus? Receptive?" Once identified, adopt that frame of mind. This preparation ensures you start with the right energy and focus.

Selecting Time and Space: Begin by using your Dowsing tool to select a quiet, comfortable space and the optimal time for your meditation. Ask your pendulum or rods, "Where is the best location in my house now (it could be a different location tomorrow) to gain the optimal benefit from my meditation? My bedroom? The den? The living room?" Continue until you get a strong 'Yes.' Then, do the same exercise for the time of day. You can even refine it further by Dowsing for a specific time within the chosen hour. Once done, you'll know you have aligned the stars for the perfect conditions for a perfect session.

Grounding and Centering: Before settling into your routine, take a few moments to ground yourself. Sit comfortably, close your eyes, and take several deep breaths. Use Mindfulness techniques to bring your awareness to the present moment, feeling the connection between your body and the earth.

Focus on the sensations of your body touching the surface beneath you—whether it's the floor, a cushion, or a chair. Feel the weight of your body and the solidity of the ground supporting you. Let this connection to the earth serve as a reminder of your rootedness and stability in the present moment.

Recall Your Intentions: Hold your pendulum and silently repeat your intentions, allowing the energy of your goals to infuse your practice. For instance, if your goal is emotional balance after a rough day, you might think, "I want to bring my emotions into balance and harmony." As you silently repeat this intention, swing your pendulum in your Yes configuration and wait until it stops. This simple ritual helps direct your energy toward a focused and purposeful meditation session.

Dowsing for Insights

Now, use your Dowsing tools to gain insights into your current state. Ask questions like, "What's my current energy level? Is it more than 60 percent?" If you get a Yes, continue refining your question until you get a precise answer. After your meditation, take the same measurements to see how the session has benefited you. This process is like having your own personal trainer, guiding you to ensure your practice is effective and meaningful.

As you move into your Mindfulness meditation, focus on your breath, bodily sensations, or a chosen focal point. Stay aware of any intuitive insights or energetic shifts, using the awareness gained from Dowsing to deepen your practice. This heightened awareness helps you tune in to your body, emotions, and mental state with greater clarity.

After the meditation, take a moment to reflect on your experience. As I said, use your Dowsing tools again to check your energy levels and validate the benefits of your session. Journaling your observations can also be helpful—note any changes, insights, or emotions that arose during the practice. Over time, these reflections will highlight patterns and guide you in refining your practice further.

Consistency and Routine

Consistency is key to deepening your practice and reaping the long-term benefits. By regularly integrating Dowsing and Mindfulness into your daily routine, you enhance both your intuitive abilities and your ability to stay present in the moment. Regular sessions allow you to build on each experience, gradually increasing the depth of your intuition and Mindfulness.

Start with manageable goals—a short session each day, or even a few minutes of breath awareness. As you progress, you can gradually increase the duration and complexity of your practice. Just as physical exercise strengthens the body over time, this combined modality strengthens both your intuition and your ability to stay grounded in the present moment.

Chapter 34

GETTING PERSONAL WITH YOUR PENDULUM

Your pendulum is a versatile tool that can help you personalize your meditation and Mindfulness practices. Before each session, you can ask questions like, "Should I focus on my breath during this session?" or "Is body scan the best technique for me today?" Use the pendulum's response to tailor your practice to your current state of mind and needs.

For example, if your pendulum indicates that a body scan is the most effective technique for that day, take time to focus on the sensations in each part of your body, from your toes to your head, observing any tension or discomfort. Allow your breath to gently soften any areas of tightness. This type of personalized guidance ensures that each session is aligned with your inner needs, making your practice more impactful.

You can also regularly use Dowsing to track your emotional state and progress. Ask questions like, "Has my stress level decreased since starting this practice?" or "Am I feeling more centered?" Tracking these changes will give you confidence that your practice is leading to tangible benefits, reinforcing your commitment.

Exploring Subconscious Blocks and Patterns

Dowsing is a powerful tool for exploring the subconscious mind, where hidden blocks and patterns may reside. You can ask, "Do I have any subconscious blocks that need addressing?" or "Is there a pattern in my behavior that I need to understand?" If the pendulum gives you a Yes, you can refine your question further, exploring the origins of these blocks or patterns.

For example, you might ask, "Are these blocks related to a specific event in my past?" or "Were these patterns established during childhood?" Continue refining your questions until you uncover the root cause of the issue. By bringing these subconscious influences into conscious awareness, you open the door to healing and transformation.

Dowsing also provides intuitive insights that can guide your self-awareness. You might ask, "Is there a specific area of my life that I need to focus on today?" or "Should I spend more time reflecting on my emotions?" These types of questions guide your attention toward areas of personal growth that require your focus *at this moment in time*, helping you uncover aspects of yourself that may have been hidden or neglected.

Tailoring Your Mindfulness Practice

Once you've gained insights through Dowsing, use this information to tailor your Mindfulness session. For instance, if Dowsing reveals heightened stress levels, you might focus on stress-relief techniques like breath awareness or visualization during your meditation. If emotional blockages are uncovered, consider incorporating loving-kindness meditation to foster healing and compassion.

On a practical level, you can also use Dowsing to help create daily meditation routines that are aligned with your energy and goals. Ask questions like, "Is today a good day for a long meditation session?" or "Is a short, focused practice more suitable for me today?" This ensures that your routines are not only effective but also flexible and responsive to your needs in the moment.

Adapting and Evolving

Your practice should evolve as you do. Regularly adapt your meditation sessions based on your intuitive feedback. Ask questions like, "Do I need to change my meditation technique today?" or "Is there a more effective way to achieve my goals?" This adaptability keeps your practice dynamic and ensures it continues to meet your needs.

You might blend traditional Mindfulness techniques with your Dowsing insights. For example, combining breath awareness with Dowsing-guided visualization can create a more powerful meditation experience. Begin by asking, "Which breathwork technique should I use today—4-7-8 breathing? Alternate nostril breathing? Box breathing?" Or "Which part of my body needs the most attention—lower half? Upper half? Head?" These insights help focus your efforts where they are most needed.

Visualization is a powerful tool in meditation, and Dowsing can help you choose the most effective imagery. You might ask, "Should I visualize a peaceful beach? A serene forest? A placid lake? A forest glade?" This targeted approach enhances the power of your visualizations, making them more impactful and aligned with your current inner needs.

Spreading a Little Loving-Kindness

Incorporate Dowsing into your **loving-kindness meditation** to personalize the practice. You could ask, "Who should I focus my loving-kindness on today—my sister? A friend? My grumpy boss?" Or "Is there someone in particular who needs my positive energy?" Swing your pendulum in your **Yes** mode and let your thoughts drift. A name or identity will float to the surface. This integration ensures that your meditation is not only meaningful but also laser-aligned with where your focus is most needed.

Addressing Challenges in Meditation

Beware the Hurdles: Restlessness and distractions can be significant challenges in meditation. Use Dowsing to identify their causes by asking, "What is causing my restlessness today—am I losing enthusiasm? Or am I just not in the mood?" or "Is there something specific distracting me—am I worried about a health issue? Is a family member in trouble?" Present relevant options to get your answer. Once identified, you can address these issues directly, improving your focus and deepening your meditation session.

Managing Stress and Anxiety: Combine Dowsing and Mindfulness to manage stress and anxiety more effectively. Ask, "What is the root cause of my anxiety today?" (provide a series of options) or "Which Mindfulness technique will help me reduce stress right now?" This integrated approach provides targeted solutions, enhancing your overall well-being and helping you tackle stress and anxiety head-on.

Resolving Emotional Blockages: Emotional blockages can hinder your progress in meditation. Identify and resolve these blockages with the help of Dowsing. Ask, "Do I have an emotional blockage related to my recent argument?" Or "What can I do to heal this emotional wound?" Supplementary Yes/No questions help you get to the heart of the matter. These insights will guide your healing process.

Reflecting on Progress and Growth

Take time to reflect on your personal growth and achievements. You might ask, "What progress have I made? On a scale of 1-100, more than 10 percent? 20 percent?" or "How has my practice transformed me? Am I calmer? Less stressed? More forgiving?" This reflection reinforces your commitment and highlights your accomplishments, motivating you to continue developing your routine.

Encourage yourself to carry on exploring and innovating within your meditation. Ask, "What new areas should I explore?" Swing your pendulum in Yes mode and allow thoughts to bubble up from your subconscious. Or, "How can I innovate my practice?" Do the same. While traditional Mindfulness focuses on internal awareness, Dowsing adds a layer of validation, giving you the confidence that you're being guided for maximum effectiveness.

Chapter 35

MAKE SENSE OF THE CHAOS WITH YOUR SECRET WEAPON

In the 'washing the dishes' example we looked at earlier, before you start you could dowse the question: "Is now a good time for a Mindfulness exercise?" If the answer is No, don't even try. Leave it for another day because your pendulum knows you're just not in the right mood. But if it's a Yes, you can start feeling 'in the moment' and enjoy the experience.

When the dishes are gleaming and stacked in the cupboard, you could dowse, "On a scale of 1-100, what level of benefit did my complete being receive from my washing-up Mindfulness? Was it more than 50%? Yes. 60%? Yes. 70%? No. 65%? No." So, you know you've benefited by more than 60%. You can get the exact figure by continuing the process of elimination.

Mindfulness has exploded onto the scene in recent years for good reason. It's all about tuning in, becoming hyper-aware of the present moment—your thoughts, feelings, the whole shebang. Adding a Dowsing element can be a total game-changer for calming a runaway mind and zoning in on the task at hand.

Think of it as a way to understand yourself and your emotions better. It can especially help during periods of major upheaval, keeping you positive and grounded. Mindfulness with Dowsing is the ultimate bridge between body and mind, a path to rebalancing your physical and emotional well-being.

Going through a massive life shift? Meditation can be your secret weapon for making sense of the chaos. By figuring out where you are and where you're headed, you gain clarity. It's about embracing the flow, resisting less, and opening yourself more, navigating change with greater ease.

Enhancing Focus and Intuition Through Dowsing Techniques

A reminder: Dowsing isn't just about finding answers; it's a powerful way to enhance your focus and intuition—crucial components of a robust Mindfulness practice. Use your pendulum to set intentions before meditation. Ask questions like, "Will this technique enhance my focus today?" or "Is this the right time for intuitive insights?" Now that you and your pendulum are good friends, feel free to ask it anything that might deepen your Mindfulness journey. In fact, make a point of meditating on the most effective questions for you.

Over time, this dual approach of Dowsing and Mindfulness will strengthen your mental clarity and intuitive abilities. You'll notice a heightened sense of awareness and an ability to trust your inner guidance more readily. This combination makes your meditation more personalized and deeply enriching.

Each person's Mindfulness needs are unique, and Dowsing can help you tailor your practice in a way that's perfect for you. Begin by identifying areas you want to explore or improve, such as reducing stress, increasing focus, or enhancing emotional balance.

You can also dowse for the duration of your sessions. Ask, "What is the ideal length for my meditation today?" This ensures you're practicing for the optimal amount of time without feeling rushed or overextended. Personalizing your Mindfulness practice with Dowsing not only makes it more effective but also keeps you attuned to your evolving needs. Here are some specific techniques:

- **Establish a Grounding Ritual:** Before embarking on any Dowsing/Mindfulness session, establish a simple ritual to ground yourself and center your energy. Take a few deep breaths, focusing on the sensation of your breath entering and leaving your body. Perhaps light a candle or burn some incense to create a calming atmosphere. This mindful ritual sets the tone for your Dowsing practice, promoting a state of present-moment awareness.

- **Focus on the Journey:** Dowsing can be a goal-oriented practice—finding a lost pet, locating a water source, or identifying detrimental energies in your home. However, it's crucial to appreciate the journey itself—especially when our goal is perfect Mindfulness! Pay attention to the subtle sensations in your body as you hold the Dowsing tool. Notice the environment around you—the sounds, the smells, the temperature.

GRATITUDE IS THE ATTITUDE

This mindful awareness of the present moment is just as valuable as the answer you ultimately receive from your Dowsing practice. By focusing on the journey, rather than just the destination, you enhance the quality of your meditation and allow yourself to fully engage with the process.

- **Embrace the Dance of the Dowsing Tool:** Forget rigid expectations! The beauty of Dowsing lies in its subtle movements. The pendulum might swing in unexpected ways, or the L-rods might twitch erratically. Instead of interpreting these movements as "wrong," approach them with curiosity. They might be offering additional information, guiding you down a path you hadn't considered. Trust the dance of the Dowsing tool, and allow it to guide your exploration of the present moment.

- **Practice Gratitude for Every Response:** Regardless of whether the Dowsing answer aligns with your initial desires, cultivate an attitude of gratitude. Thank your intuition for its guidance and for offering insights you might not have considered otherwise. This practice of gratitude reinforces the connection between your conscious mind and your intuition, fostering a deeper state of Mindfulness and acceptance.

Chapter 36

DON'T FORGET...

• **Slow Down and Be Present:** Take your time, formulate your questions with care, and observe the world around you with a sense of curiosity.

• **Embrace the Mystery:** Dowsing isn't about achieving absolute certainty. It's about opening yourself to possibilities and trusting your intuition. Embrace the mystery of the unseen forces that guide your Dowsing practice.

• **Let Go of Attachment to Outcomes:** Don't become fixated on a specific answer from your Dowsing tool. Approach each session with an open mind and a willingness to accept whatever guidance arises. You'll know when you're getting an accurate answer—it'll often be one you're not expecting!

By integrating these Mindfulness techniques and cultivating a mindful Dowsing mindset, you'll unlock a treasure trove of benefits. You'll find yourself becoming more present in everyday moments, making decisions with greater clarity, and connecting with a deeper sense of intuition that guides you on your life's journey.

Building a Sustainable Practice – some reminders

• **Daily Routine:** Integrate short Dowsing and Mindfulness sessions into your daily routine. Start with just five minutes each morning or evening and build up from there.

• **Track Progress:** Use a journal to record your findings and progress. Note how you feel before and after meditation, and any insights gained.

• **Stay Flexible:** Adjust your practices based on Dowsing feedback. If something isn't working, don't hesitate to try a different approach.

• **Guided Visualizations:** Use Dowsing to choose the most effective visualization exercises. For instance, ask, "Which visualization will help me feel more relaxed—peaceful forest glade? Tropical beach? A sacred site?"

• **Deep Relaxation Techniques:** Dowse for methods that enhance relaxation and stress relief. Techniques like progressive muscle relaxation or guided imagery can be particularly effective.

• **Stay Open and Curious:** Mindfulness and Dowsing are both practices of exploration. Approach each session with a sense of curiosity and openness.

• **Trust Your Intuition:** If something feels off, trust your gut. Dowsing is a guide, but your intuition is the ultimate authority.

• **Be Patient:** Like any skill, it takes practice. Be patient with yourself as you learn and refine your technique.

AND THIS...

• **Calibrate Your Pendulum:** Hold it steady and ask basic questions to ensure it responds correctly. For example, ask, "Is my name [your name]?" to confirm the 'Yes' response, and "Is my name [not your name]?" for the 'No' response.

• **Set Intentions:** Clearly state your goal for the meditation session. For instance, "I want this meditation session to clear my anger from being bullied by my boss today."

• **Dowse for Timing:** Ask the pendulum to determine the best time and duration for meditation. For example, "Is 6 AM a good time for meditation?" Observe the response and adjust accordingly.

• **Choose Your Technique:** Dowse to select the most beneficial meditation technique for the day. Ask, "Should I practice breath awareness today?" or "Is body scan meditation best for today?"

- **Morning Check-In:** Use your pendulum to assess your energy levels and choose a focus for the day. Ask, "What is my current energy level on a scale of 1 to 100?" and "What should I focus on today to maintain positive energy?" (Provide a series of Yes/No options.)

- **Midday Pause:** Dowse for a quick Mindfulness exercise to re-energize. Ask, "What can I do right now to boost my energy and focus?" Again, offer several options.

- **Evening Reflection:** Ask your pendulum to guide you in reflecting on your day and planning for tomorrow. For example, ask, "What was the most significant lesson of my day?" or "How can I improve tomorrow?" Offer possibilities, and let the pendulum guide you.

By incorporating Dowsing into your Mindfulness practice, you can tailor your meditation to the times when you are most receptive, creating a more effective and enriching experience. Keep exploring, stay curious, and let your pendulum become an extension of your intuition.

LOCATING THOSE BLOCKAGES

To locate energy blockages, start by relaxing and holding your pendulum. Ask, "Do I have any energy blockages in my body right now?" If the response is 'Yes,' proceed with more specific questions like, "Is the blockage in my head?" If 'No,' move to other areas of the body until you find the location. Once identified, use guided imagery to visualize the blockage clearing. Imagine a healing light dissolving the blockage, restoring the energy flow.

- **Combining Dowsing with Chakra Meditation:** Dowse to determine which chakras need attention. Ask your pendulum,

"Which chakra should I focus on today?" Once identified, meditate by visualizing that chakra's color and energy, using affirmations like, "My [specific chakra] is balanced and strong and will remain strong for as long as is appropriate." This practice enhances the flow of energy through your body's energy centers.

• **Dowsing for Intuitive Insights During Meditation:** Before meditating, set your pendulum in search mode and ask what insights you should seek. Questions like, "What personal issue should I focus on today?" or "What aspect of my life needs clarity?" Then swing your pendulum into its positive (Yes) mode and allow it to guide your thoughts. This focused approach can help uncover deeper truths and intuitive knowledge.

Final Thoughts on Your Mindfulness Journey

Now that you can trust your pendulum or rods, ask, "What is my appropriate state of mind to achieve the optimum benefit from my meditation? Calmness? Alert focus? Receptive?" Once identified, adopt that frame of mind.

More on Guided Imagery: Mindfulness often incorporates guided imagery to cultivate specific emotions or states. Before visualization, dowse different calming or focus-enhancing words or phrases. Choose the one that elicits the strongest positive response from your tool, and use it as the 'anchor' for your visualization.

For instance, you might be conjuring up images of a Caribbean beach, the sand under your feet, and the sun setting beyond an azure sea. So phrases like 'relax,' 'stillness,' 'tranquil,' 'peaceful,' or 'serenity' might come to mind. Take time to dowse which word or phrase would be the most effective at this moment (it could be totally different for another occasion) and repeat it often during your session. Are you beginning to see how Dowsing supercharges your meditation? It ensures you have the optimum experience every time. As Dowsing becomes an automatic part of your daily life, you will find your own ways of using it to enhance your life.

Dowsing for Optimal Meditation Duration

Finding the perfect meditation length can be a personal journey. Dowsing can help you discover the best duration. Before you begin, ask your Dowsing tool something like, "Show me the perfect length of time for this Mindfulness session—is it more than 20 minutes?" If 'No,' then, "Is it more than 15 minutes?" If 'Yes,' "Is it 16 minutes?" And so on, until you have a precise duration. This method will help you identify the point where the effectiveness of the meditation begins to diminish, ensuring you get the most out of your practice.

Dowsing for Post-Meditation Integration

Mindfulness isn't just about what happens on the meditation mat. Dowsing can help bridge the gap between practice and daily life. After your session, dowse for activities that will best integrate your newfound sense of calm or focus into your day. This could involve spending time in nature, journaling, or engaging in a creative pursuit. For instance, you could ask, "What will help me maintain this feeling of peace throughout the day?" Dowse for options, and let the pendulum guide you towards the right action.

Important Considerations

At all times, remember that mindful awareness is your primary focus, with Dowsing as a complementary guide. If a Dowsing response feels off, don't force it. Dowsing can be a deeply personal experience, so give yourself the space to experiment and find what works best for you. And never forget the cardinal rule: practice, practice, practice!

Now that we have explored the fascinating worlds of Dowsing and Mindfulness, and have discovered how these tools can amplify your intuition, it's time to truly bridge these two modalities. Go for it and discover a more mindful and serene life.

Chapter 37

THIS IS REAL LIFE

Let's dive into a few case studies from people who've trodden this path before you, combining Dowsing with Mindfulness to create real and lasting change.

Sarah's Journey to Inner Balance

Background:

Sarah, a 42-year-old professional living in Seattle, found herself struggling with chronic stress and anxiety due to her demanding job. Despite trying various Mindfulness techniques, she felt something was missing from her practice. While researching alternative methods to enhance her mental and emotional well-being, she stumbled upon Dowsing. Intrigued, Sarah decided to combine Dowsing with her Mindfulness routine to see if it could bring the balance she was desperately seeking.

Challenges and Approach:

Initially, Sarah struggled with skepticism. Although she was open-minded, the idea of using a pendulum or rods to guide her practice seemed far-fetched. She also found it challenging to trust the answers she received through Dowsing, often second-guessing whether she was subconsciously influencing the outcome. Additionally, Sarah had difficulty integrating Dowsing into her fast-paced lifestyle. Finding the time and mental space to practice both disciplines consistently was a significant hurdle.

How She Overcame These Hurdles:

To conquer her skepticism, Sarah decided to approach Dowsing as an experiment rather than as a definitive solution. She began by using the pendulum to answer simple, low-pressure questions unrelated to her Mindfulness practice—questions like what time to eat lunch or which book to read next. As she started seeing accurate and beneficial results, her confidence in Dowsing grew.

To integrate Dowsing with Mindfulness, Sarah simplified her approach. Instead of setting aside extra time for Dowsing, she incorporated it into her existing routine. Before each meditation session, she would dowse to determine the best time to meditate, the focus of her session, and even which Mindfulness technique to use. This method allowed her to practice both disciplines without feeling overwhelmed.

Results and Transformation:

As Sarah continued her combined practice, she noticed a profound shift in her well-being. Dowsing helped her tailor her Mindfulness sessions to her specific needs each day, making them more effective. For instance, on days when she felt particularly anxious, the pendulum would guide her toward meditation techniques that calmed her nerves, such as deep breathing or guided visualization.

Over time, Sarah's anxiety levels significantly decreased. She felt more in control of her emotions and better equipped to handle stress. The practice also deepened her self-awareness, helping her uncover subconscious blocks that had been contributing to her anxiety. Through regular Dowsing and Mindfulness, Sarah transformed her life, achieving a balance and inner peace that had previously eluded her.

Key Takeaways from Sarah's Experience

You may have noticed that Sarah did not discover a quick fix. It took her months of persistence, tenacity, and self-discipline, but the rewards were worth it. Here are a few key techniques Sarah used, which could be helpful for you:

Optimal Meditation Timing: Sarah found that Dowsing for the best time to meditate helped her avoid periods when she was likely to be distracted or fatigued. As a result, her meditation sessions became more focused and rewarding. By meditating at the times when her energy was naturally aligned, she found it easier to enter a deep state of Mindfulness.

Choosing the Right Mindfulness Technique: Before beginning her practice, Sarah would dowse for the most appropriate Mindfulness technique for that day. For example, she would ask, "Should I focus on breath awareness today?" or "Is loving-kindness meditation the best approach for me right now?" By allowing her pendulum to guide her, Sarah was able to choose techniques that resonated with her current emotional and mental state, leading to a more effective practice.

Measuring Energy Levels: Sarah used Dowsing to check her energy levels before and after meditation. This allowed her to measure the tangible benefits of her sessions. She would ask, "Is my energy level above 70 percent?" and make adjustments based on the response. After her session, she would dowse again to see the percentage change, which often validated the effectiveness of her meditation.

And What Were the Key Lessons Sarah Learned That Would Be Useful to You?

Start Simple

This helped to build her confidence. Beginning with basic Yes/No questions allowed Sarah to trust the process and sharpen her Dowsing skills. This foundation made it easier for her to apply

Dowsing to more complex decisions within her Mindfulness practice.

Be Consistent

Sarah discovered that consistency in both Dowsing and Mindfulness was crucial for seeing results. Even on days when she felt skeptical or tired, maintaining her routine reinforced her commitment and led to cumulative benefits. Regular practice helped her develop a deeper intuitive connection, making the Dowsing process more natural and accurate over time.

Trust Your Intuition

A significant part of integrating Dowsing and Mindfulness is learning to trust your intuition. Sarah initially struggled with this, but as she continued her practice, she realized that her intuition was a reliable guide. Dowsing served as a tool to amplify this inner voice, helping her make decisions that were in tune with her true needs.

Stay Open and Flexible

Sarah learned to stay open and flexible in her practice. She didn't rigidly adhere to the results of her Dowsing but used them as a guide. If something didn't feel right during her Mindfulness session, she allowed herself to adapt and change course. This flexibility prevented frustration and kept her sessions dynamic and responsive.

Reflect and Adjust

Regular reflection on her meditation was another best practice Sarah adopted. By journaling her experiences, she could track her progress, notice patterns, and make necessary adjustments. This reflection helped her fine-tune her approach, ensuring that she continued to grow and benefit from her unorthodox approach.

Conclusion: Sarah's journey illustrates the transformative potential of combining the twin protocols of Dowsing and Mindfulness. By overcoming challenges, staying consistent, and trusting her intuition, she was able to achieve a balance and inner peace that had previously seemed out of reach. Her experiences, along with the practical examples and lessons learned, offer valuable insights for anyone looking to enhance their meditation practice.

Chapter 38

HOW JAMES TRANSFORMED HIS WORKPLACE PERFORMANCE

Background

James, a 35-year-old software engineer from San Francisco, was struggling with focus and productivity at work. He often felt overwhelmed by the fast-paced environment and tight deadlines, which led to frequent mistakes and a lack of confidence in his abilities. James had tried Mindfulness meditation before but found it challenging to maintain a consistent practice. After attending a workshop on Dowsing, he became curious about how it could enhance his focus and productivity at work.

Initial Challenges

At first James was hesitant to introduce Dowsing into his professional life. He feared that if he confided in colleagues they might view it as unscientific or strange. Moreover, he had difficulty trusting the Dowsing responses, particularly in the context of work-related decisions. Integrating these practices into his already busy schedule was another significant challenge.

Application of Techniques

Morning Focus Sessions: James began his workday with a brief Mindfulness session, followed by Dowsing to prioritize his tasks. He would ask questions like, "Which task should I focus on first today to maximize productivity?" Or "Is this project a priority over the others?" This helped him approach his workload with a clearer focus and better time management.

Midday Check-Ins: To maintain productivity throughout the day, James used Dowsing to determine when he needed a rest. He would ask, "Do I need a break now to restore focus?" Then he used Mindfulness techniques, such as mindful walking or deep breathing to recharge.

Decision-Making: James applied Dowsing to help with decision-making at work, particularly in high-pressure situations. For example, before making a critical coding choice, he would dowse to assess whether it was the right time or if he needed more information. This approach allowed him to make more thoughtful and confident decisions.

Results Achieved: Within a few months, James saw a marked improvement in his focus and productivity. He was completing tasks more efficiently and with fewer errors, which boosted his confidence. His colleagues noticed the change, and he began to receive positive feedback from his supervisors. The integration of Dowsing and Mindfulness into his daily routine not only enhanced his work performance but also reduced his overall stress levels. James found that he was better able to handle the pressures of his job and approach challenges with a calm, focused mindset.

HOW EMILY FOUND EMOTIONAL HEALING
Background

Emily, a 28-year-old artist from New York, had been dealing with unresolved emotional trauma from her childhood. This trauma manifested in her adult life as difficulties in relationships, frequent bouts of depression, and a general sense of disconnection from herself and others. Despite trying various forms of therapy, she felt that something was missing in her healing process. Emily discovered Dowsing through a friend and decided to explore how it could be combined with Mindfulness to address her deep-seated issues.

Initial Challenges

Emily was emotionally sensitive, and the idea of delving into her past through Dowsing felt intimidating. "What if I uncover something I'm not ready to face?" She wondered. She also struggled with the consistency of her Mindfulness practice, often feeling too overwhelmed to meditate regularly. "I don't even know if I can sit still long enough to focus on this," she thought. Additionally, Emily had doubts about whether Dowsing could provide the clarity she was seeking in her emotional healing journey. "Will this really work for something so deep?" She questioned.

Identifying Emotional Blockages: Emily began by using Dowsing to uncover the root causes of her emotional distress. She would ask questions like, "Is my current depression linked to childhood trauma?" Or "Do I have unresolved feelings about my relationship with my parents?" After identifying specific issues, she used Mindfulness practices, such as loving-kindness meditation and body scan, to process and release these emotions.

Daily Emotional Check-Ins: Emily incorporated daily Mindfulness and Dowsing check-ins to monitor her emotional state. "What is my emotional state this morning?" She would ask, or "Do I need to focus on self-compassion today?" Based on the responses, she tailored her Mindfulness practice to address her emotional needs. "If my pendulum says self-compassion, that's what I'll work on today," she thought.

Guided Visualizations: Emily used Dowsing to guide her visualization meditations, asking questions like, "What should I visualize to heal my inner self?" Or "Which memory do I need to revisit for healing?" These guided visualizations became a powerful tool for her emotional recovery, helping her reconnect with, and heal, her past. "This feels right; I'm finally starting to understand myself better," she noted in her journal.

Results Achieved

Over time, Emily experienced profound emotional healing and self-discovery. She noticed a significant reduction in her depressive episodes and felt a stronger connection to herself and others. "It's like I've lifted a heavy weight off my heart," she reflected. By regularly using Dowsing to guide her Mindfulness practice, Emily gained a deeper understanding of her emotional landscape and learned how to navigate it with compassion and resilience. This integration of Dowsing and Mindfulness not only facilitated her healing process but also empowered her to embrace her emotional sensitivity as a source of strength and creativity.

Conclusions

These case studies illustrate how integrating Dowsing and Mindfulness can lead to significant improvements in various areas of life, from managing anxiety and improving work performance to emotional healing and self-discovery. Each individual faced unique challenges but found success by applying these techniques in a way that resonated with their personal needs and circumstances. Their stories demonstrate the transformative potential of combining both practices for personal growth and well-being.

Now You've Completed Your Journey and learned a unique Mindfulness/Dowsing protocol, here are a few real-life applications (I'm sure by now you could add a lot more) to stimulate your creative thinking:

Mindfulness and Dowsing in the Workplace

Mindful Task Selection: At the start of your workday, use your Dowsing tool to prioritize tasks. For example, you could ask, "Which task should I focus on first to maximize productivity?" Or "Is now the best time to work on this project?" This helps ensure that you're tackling the most important tasks when your energy and focus are at their peak.

Mindfulness Breaks: Take short Mindfulness breaks throughout the day. Use a pendulum to determine when a rest is needed by asking, "Is now a good time for a Mindfulness break?" During the break, practice mindful breathing or a short meditation to clear your mind and recharge your focus.

Managing Stress: If you feel overwhelmed, pause and ask your pendulum, "What is the source of my stress?" Or "How can I reduce my stress right now?" Use the answer to guide your next steps, whether that means taking a walk, practicing deep breathing, or addressing a specific task.

Chapter 39

IF YOU'VE GOT THIS FAR – YOU'RE ALMOST QUALIFIED, BUT DON'T FORGET...

Before making important decisions, use Mindfulness to clear your mind of distractions. Then, ask your Dowsing tool, "Is this the right choice for me?" Or "Should I proceed with this decision now?" This can help ensure that your choices are made with clarity and alignment with your goals.

Balancing Workloads: If you're juggling multiple projects, dowse to assess where to allocate your time and energy. For instance, ask, "Which project needs my attention most today?" Or "How should I balance my workload to reduce stress?"

Mindful Listening: In conversations with others, practice mindful listening by fully focusing on the speaker without planning your response. Before engaging in a potentially challenging conversation, dowse to check your emotional readiness by asking, "Am I in the right state of mind for this discussion?"

Resolving Conflicts: Use Dowsing to gain insights into underlying issues during a conflict. For example, ask, "What is the root cause of this disagreement?" Or "How can I approach this situation with compassion?" Mindfulness can then be used to stay present and calm during the conversation, preventing reactive responses.

Setting Boundaries: Before discussing boundaries with someone, use Mindfulness to reflect on your needs. Then, ask your

Dowsing tool, "Is this the right time to set this boundary?" Or "How can I communicate my needs effectively?"

Mindful Presence: Practice being fully present with your loved ones by engaging in Mindfulness exercises together, such as mindful breathing or walking. Use Dowsing to enhance these practices by asking, "What activity will strengthen our connection today?" Or "How can I best support my partner emotionally?"

Showing Appreciation: Use Dowsing to guide you in showing appreciation for others. For instance, ask, "What gesture of appreciation will be most meaningful to my partner/friend/family member?" This can help you express gratitude in a way that resonates deeply with them.

Choosing Healthy Habits: Use Dowsing to select the best health practices for your current needs. For example, ask, "Should I focus on improving my diet or increasing my physical activity?" Or "What exercise will benefit my body most today?" Follow up with Mindfulness practices, such as mindful eating or mindful movement, to enhance the effectiveness of these habits.

Managing Energy Levels: Dowse to check your energy levels throughout the day. Ask, "Is my energy level above 70%?" Or "Do I need to rest or recharge now?" Use Mindfulness techniques, such as deep breathing or a short meditation, to restore energy when needed.

Mindful Eating: Before meals, practice mindful eating by Dowsing to choose the most nourishing foods for your body. Ask, "What type of food will best support my health right now?" Or "Should I eat this meal now or wait until later?" During the meal, engage in Mindfulness by savoring each bite, noticing the flavors, textures, and aromas.

Mindful Stress Reduction: When feeling stressed, use Dowsing to identify the source of your stress and the best way to alleviate it. For instance, ask, "What is causing my anxiety?" Or "What Mindfulness practice will help me feel calmer right now?" Engage in the recommended practice, such as a body scan meditation or deep breathing exercise, to reduce stress.

Enhancing Sleep Quality: Dowse to assess your readiness for sleep by asking, "Is my mind calm enough for sleep?" Or "Should I meditate before bed to improve my sleep?" Practice Mindfulness techniques, such as progressive muscle relaxation or focused breathing, to prepare your body and mind for restful sleep.

Emotional Healing: Use Dowsing to identify emotional blockages or unresolved issues. Ask, "Is there an emotion I need to process?" Or "What can I do to heal this emotional pain?" Follow up with Mindfulness practices, such as journaling, meditation, or self-compassion exercises, to support emotional healing.

Real-Life Applications:

At Work

Scenario: You're feeling overwhelmed by a project deadline.

Mindfulness: Take a few minutes to practice deep breathing, focusing on each inhale and exhale to calm your mind.

Dowsing: Ask, "What is the most effective next step to move this project forward?" Use the response to guide your immediate actions, helping you to focus and reduce stress.

In Relationships

Scenario: You need to have a difficult conversation with a partner or colleague.

Mindfulness: Before the conversation, practice a short Mindfulness exercise to center yourself and approach the discussion calmly.

Dowsing: Ask, "How can I communicate my concerns most effectively?" Or "What should I avoid saying to prevent escalation?" This ensures that your approach is thoughtful and aligned with your intentions.

For Health

Scenario: You're feeling low energy and unsure if you should exercise or rest.

Mindfulness: Pause and check in with your body through a brief body scan meditation.

Dowsing: Ask, "Will exercising improve my energy levels?" Or "Do I need rest more than exercise right now?" Use the response to guide your decision, ensuring that you're honoring your body's needs.

Conclusion

Integrating Mindfulness and Dowsing into your daily life can lead to profound improvements in your work, relationships, and health. By using these practices together, you can make more informed decisions, reduce stress, enhance communication, and cultivate a deeper sense of well-being. The key is to approach each aspect of life with a mindful awareness, using Dowsing as a tool to guide your actions and decisions with greater clarity and intention.

So, now you have all you need to transform your life into the "You" you always wanted to be.

Go for it!

Recommended Reading List

Dowsing

"Dowse Your Way to Psychic Power: The Ultimate Short-cut to Other Dimensions" by Anthony Talmage

Summary: In this book, Anthony Talmage provides a comprehensive guide to using Dowsing as a powerful tool for accessing other dimensions and enhancing psychic abilities. The book is filled with practical exercises, case studies, and insights that help readers tap into their intuitive potential and explore the unseen world around them.

"The Diviner's Handbook: A Guide to the Ancient Art of Dowsing" by Tom Graves

Summary: This guide explores the history, techniques, and applications of Dowsing. Tom Graves offers practical advice for both beginners and experienced dowsers, covering topics such as locating water, minerals, and lost objects, as well as exploring Dowsing's spiritual dimensions.

"Dowsing: A Journey Beyond Our Five Senses" by Hamish Miller

Summary: Renowned dowser Hamish Miller shares his experiences and insights into the practice of Dowsing. He delves into the connection between Dowsing and the spiritual world, offering readers a deeper understanding of how Dowsing can be used for personal growth and spiritual exploration.

"The Complete Guide to Dowsing: The Divining Rods and How to Use Them" by George Applegate

Summary: George Applegate provides a thorough introduction to the practice of Dowsing with rods. The book includes practical exercises and tips for developing Dowsing skills, as well as fascinating case studies that illustrate the power of Dowsing in various real-life situations.

"Letter to Robin: A Mini-Course in Pendulum Dowsing" by Walt Woods

Summary: This booklet is a practical and easy-to-follow guide to pendulum Dowsing. Written in a conversational style, it serves as an excellent introduction for beginners and includes exercises to help readers develop their Dowsing abilities.

Mindfulness and Meditation

"Wherever You Go, There You Are: Mindfulness Meditation in Everyday Life" by Jon Kabat-Zinn

Summary: Jon Kabat-Zinn introduces readers to the practice of Mindfulness meditation in this accessible and practical guide. The book emphasizes the importance of bringing Mindfulness into everyday activities and offers techniques for cultivating a mindful presence.

"The Miracle of Mindfulness: An Introduction to the Practice of Meditation" by Thich Nhat Hanh

Summary: Zen master Thich Nhat Hanh presents Mindfulness as a way of life. Through simple exercises and profound insights, he teaches readers how to develop Mindfulness in all aspects of life, from breathing and walking to working and eating.

"Radical Acceptance: Embracing Your Life With the Heart of a Buddha" by Tara Brach

Summary: Tara Brach explores the concept of radical acceptance in this transformative book. She combines Mindfulness with self-compassion to help readers overcome feelings of inadequacy and embrace their true selves.

"The Power of Now: A Guide to Spiritual Enlightenment" by Eckhart Tolle

Summary: Eckhart Tolle's book focuses on the importance of living in the present moment. Through practical exercises and spiritual insights, Tolle teaches readers how to transcend the mind's constant chatter and achieve a state of deep inner peace.

"Mindfulness in Plain English" by Bhante Henepola Gunaratana

Summary: This straightforward and practical guide to Mindfulness meditation is ideal for beginners. Bhante Gunaratana offers clear instructions on how to meditate, along with insights into the challenges and benefits of a regular Mindfulness practice.

Spirituality and Metaphysics

"The Field: The Quest for the Secret Force of the Universe" by Lynne McTaggart

Summary: Lynne McTaggart explores the concept of the "Zero Point Field," an underlying energy field that connects all things. Drawing on scientific research and metaphysical insights, McTaggart delves into the implications of this field for consciousness, healing, and the interconnectedness of life.

"The Hidden Messages in Water" by Masaru Emoto

Summary: Masaru Emoto's research into the effects of thoughts and emotions on water crystals has profound implications for understanding the power of intention and consciousness. This book presents his findings and explores how our thoughts can influence the physical world.

"The Celestine Prophecy" by James Redfield

Summary: This novel blends adventure with spiritual insights, exploring the idea that coincidences and synchronicities are meaningful events that guide us on our spiritual journey. It offers readers a narrative that encourages a deeper understanding of life's purpose and the spiritual forces at play.

Practical Guides and Exercises
"The Mindful Way Workbook: An 8-Week Program to Free Yourself from Depression and Emotional Distress" by John Teasdale, Mark Williams, and Zindel Segal

Summary: This workbook provides a step-by-step guide to practicing Mindfulness to overcome depression and emotional distress. The exercises and meditations are based on the authors' successful Mindfulness-Based Cognitive Therapy (MBCT) program.

"Dowsing for Beginners: How to Find Water, Wealth, & Lost Objects" by Richard Webster

Summary: Richard Webster's book is a practical guide for those new to Dowsing. It covers the basics of using Dowsing tools, finding water and lost objects, and using Dowsing in daily life. The book also includes exercises to help beginners develop their skills.

"The Wisdom of Insecurity: A Message for an Age of Anxiety" by Alan Watts

Summary: Alan Watts, a philosopher known for interpreting and popularizing Eastern philosophy for Western audiences, discusses how embracing uncertainty and living fully in the present moment can lead to a more meaningful and less stressful life.

A WORD FROM THE AUTHOR

If you have enjoyed this book please consider writing a review (even if it's not a good one!) and give your thoughts on social media. If you believe the book is worth sharing, please take a few seconds to let your friends know about it. Much of this book is based on the functions of our amazing conscious and unconscious human minds which have long been a fascination to me. I have learned that while science, medicine, and technology have accomplished remarkable feats, human consciousness is a powerhouse capable of delivering miracles beyond our imagination.

I cover all aspects of this in the other four books in my "Psychic Mind" series. These are *Dowse Your Way To Psychic Power*, *In Tune With The Infinite Mind*, *Unlock The Psychic Powers of Your Unconscious Mind* and *How To Crack The Cosmic Code (And plug into the hidden powers of your unconscious mind)* all available in ebook and printed versions from all good on-line bookstores.

Don't miss out!

Visit the website below and you can sign up to receive emails whenever Anthony Talmage publishes a new book. There's no charge and no obligation.

https://books2read.com/r/B-A-UVRM-FHDHF

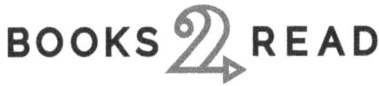

BOOKS 2 READ

Connecting independent readers to independent writers.

Did you love *Mindfulness And The Pendulum*? Then you should read *How To Crack The Cosmic Code- And Plug Into The Hidden Powers Of Your Unconscious Mind*[1] by Anthony Talmage!

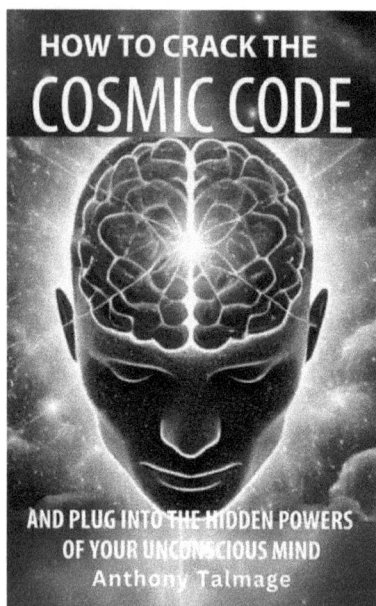

Do you ever feel stuck in a routine, as if life has lost its magic? *How to Crack the Cosmic Code* is your invitation to break free. Imagine tapping into a hidden power—a force that connects you to the universe itself, one that can help you reach your goals, reshape reality, and discover meaning in the everyday.

In this transformative guide, author Anthony Talmage reveals how the human mind is more than we've been taught. Think of it as a gateway to the Cosmic Consciousness, an infinite database of wisdom and possibility. Through insights drawn from ancient teachings and modern discoveries, you'll uncover tools to unlock your intuition, connect with universal knowledge, and explore the mystery of consciousness.

Whether you're looking to overcome obstacles, redefine your purpose, or glimpse the extraordinary potential within you, *How to Crack the Cosmic Code* shows you how to use your mind as a powerful ally. This isn't just a book; it's an experience designed to change how you see the world—and your place within it. Prepare to step into a life of wonder and possibility.

Read more at https://www.facebook.com.

Also by Anthony Talmage

Psychic Mind series
Dowse Your Way To Psychic Power
In Tune With The Infinite Mind
Unlock The Psychic Powers Of Your Unconsious Mind
Mindfulness And The Pendulum
Mindfulness And The Pendulum

Standalone
Cut To The Quick-Short Stories For Busy People
How To Crack The Cosmic Code- And Plug Into The Hidden
Powers Of Your Unconscious Mind
Kingdom And The Glory
The Kirov Conspiracy
Ticket To A Killing

Watch for more at https://www.facebook.com.

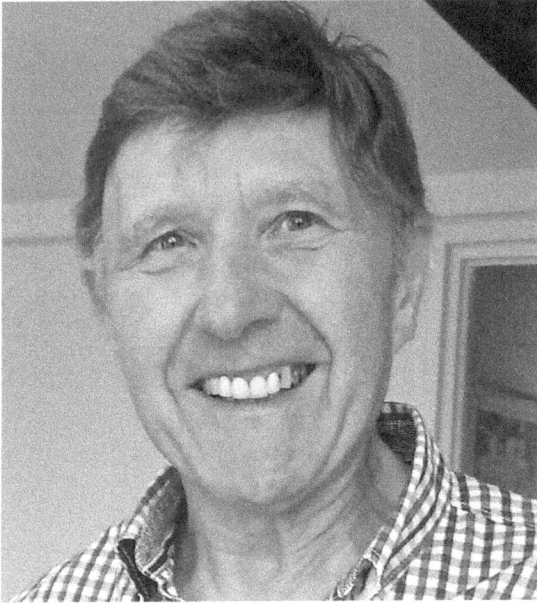

About the Author

In his career as a BBC journalist and broadcaster and a national and regional journalist, Anthony Talmage had written his fair share of stories about The Unexplained, which is what prompted him to develop his interest in the paranormal. It led him to membership of the widely-respected Society for Psychical Research, and the British Society of Dowsers where he learned the art of divining. After establishing the Guernsey Society of Dowsers, he went on to focus his dowsing skills on the areas of Health and Subtle Energies. He later taught dowsing at the Guernsey College of Further Education and he still runs workshops on both dowsing and energy healing. Through all his many years of researching the metaphysical, esoteric, mystical, occult, paranormal, the Mysterious and Things That Go Bump in the Night Anthony came to the conclusion that The Unconscious Mind is the one factor common to them all. Which, he believes, means that everyone has access to psychic or so-called paranormal powers. This is now his mission – to encourage everyone to use their sixth sense to fulfil their potential.

Read more at https://www.facebook.com.

Milton Keynes UK
Ingram Content Group UK Ltd.
UKHW041816151124
451262UK00005B/588

9 798224 015962